FIGHT CANCER

Professor Karol Sikora and
Dr Hilary Thomas

BBC BOOKS

Published by BBC Books,
a division of BBC Enterprises Limited,
Woodlands, 80 Wood Lane, London W12 0TT
First published 1989

ISBN 0 563 20863 5

Set in 10½/13 pt Janson by Ace Filmsetting Ltd, Frome, Somerset
Printed and bound in Great Britain by Redwood Burn Ltd, Trowbridge, Wilts.
Cover printed by Fletchers of Norwich

Contents

Karol Sikora PhD, FRCR, FRCP is Professor of Clinical Oncology (Cancer Medicine) at the Royal Postgraduate Medical School, Hammersmith Hospital, London. He studied medicine at Cambridge and the Middlesex Hospital and after working as a junior doctor in several London hospitals went back to Cambridge to do research in the MRC Laboratory for Molecular Biology. He then spent a year at Stanford in California where he saw how a major US cancer centre operated. On returning he set up the Ludwig Institute for Cancer Research in Cambridge before taking up his present position in 1986. He is accredited in both radiotherapy and medical oncology and feels strongly that cancer care is best given in centres of excellence where expertise can be concentrated. His main research involves the application of modern molecular biology to cancer treatment. In his department at Hammersmith there is a large Imperial Cancer Research Fund group exploring the factors that cause cancer cells to grow and multiply. He is the author of over a hundred papers in the medical literature, ten books and co-editor of a leading textbook for specialists – *The Treatment of Cancer*. He is married with three children.

Hilary Thomas MA, MB, MRCP is twenty-nine and studied medicine at New Hall, Cambridge. Her clinical training was at University College Hospital, London. As a medical student she travelled extensively, spending three months studying the nutrition of village children in the Gambia and working in a leper colony in Andhrapradesh. After qualifying she trained in general medicine, obtaining the MRCP in 1987. She then specialised in oncology, an aim she had pursued steadily since a student. She is currently a registrar in clinical oncology at the Royal Postgraduate Medical School, Hammersmith Hospital. She is leading a project involving the clinical investigation of several new cancer therapies. In what spare time she has, she is active in the Medical Women's Federation which seeks to improve career opportunities for women in medicine.

CANCER –
THE DISEASE

Cancer is a common problem. One in three of us will develop it. We read about it daily in newspapers and magazines. It seems to be all round us, gathering momentum. Even in the late 1980s, when much is taken for granted and patients are more likely to be fully informed, the association between cancer and death is so strong that the topic may remain taboo. It is a myth that everyone with cancer will eventually die from it. Many people, particularly if the disease is diagnosed at an early stage, make a complete recovery. Indeed, the death rate for many chronic medical conditions is far greater than that of cancer.

Moreover, in the last twenty years there have been dramatic strides in our understanding of what cancer is and how best to treat it. Cancers that were almost uniformly fatal in the past, such as Hodgkin's disease and testicular cancer, are nearly completely curable now. There have been tremendous improvements in the care of all cancer patients, from making the diagnosis with greater precision to following what is happening during treatment and controlling any unpleasant symptoms. We have much better information on the numbers and sort of people it is likely to affect. It is not really getting much commoner – it's just that we live longer and cancer occurs more commonly in the very old. We have also managed to break through some of the taboos that used to surround cancer – so the diagnosis is quite open between doctor and patient and between family and friends. But this new frankness means that the need for information has never been greater. Consumerism has hit health care in a big way. If used correctly it can change for the better the way we live. But to avoid tilting at windmills it must be based on facts. Here we provide an unbiased guide through the world of cancer and its treatment. A greater understanding will dispel many myths and show the promising path forward.

CELLS AND CANCER

To understand what cancer is, we must look at how our body is made. We are all built of cells so tiny they are only visible down a powerful microscope. About one thousand billion are needed to make a person. The cells of different tissues are specialised to have different functions. A muscle cell has tiny molecular ropes to allow it to contract; a skin cell a tough waterproof coat to protect us from the environment and a liver cell a little chemical refinery continuously cleaning the blood of potential poisons. In most people, these different cells are working in perfect harmony. But sometimes they can go wrong. If a single cell dies, one of its many identical partners simply takes over its job. But if a cell starts to grow and divide in an abnormal way, then problems can arise. To explain this, we need to look first at how normal cells grow and reproduce.

Normal cell structure and growth

Normal cells consist of a membrane, cytoplasm and a nucleus (see illustration opposite). The **membrane** is a complex structure which includes a number of large protein molecules stretching across it. These project an external portion – which acts as a receptor, and an internal portion. Signals received by the external part are transmitted through the membrane, so telling the cell what to do. When we are suddenly frightened, for example, adrenaline is released into the bloodstream. The cell receptors pick this up and prepare our muscles and nervous system to deal rapidly with the situation. Cell surface markers also enable the body's immune system to recognise foreign molecules or infected cells – processes which are vital in resisting and overcoming infections. In addition, the cell membrane provides a 'skeleton' for the cell and helps to maintain the correct balance of chemicals inside.

The **cytoplasm** is the 'biological soup' inside the cell which contains structures involved in how the cell works and grows. These are vital for the division of the cell into two daughter cells during growth and for the production of substances by the cell as part of its everyday function.

The nucleus contains material known as DNA (deoxyribonucleic acid) – a chemical sequence in which information which is passed on from one cell to the next (and indeed from one generation to the next) is stored. It is this information which determines whether, for example, a cell will be a specialised muscle cell or a skin cell. It is also through the DNA that physical characteristics – height, colour of hair and eyes, and so on – are passed on from parents to children.

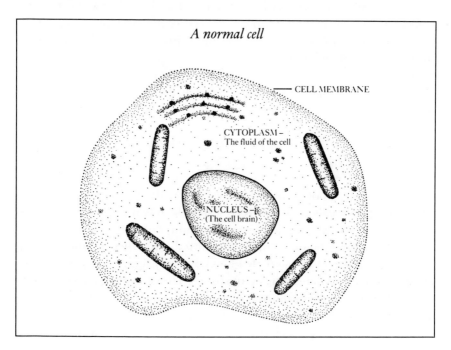

A normal cell

CELL MEMBRANE

CYTOPLASM –
The fluid of the cell

NUCLEUS –
(The cell brain)

All complex organisms, man included, grow from a single cell by a series of events in which a cell splits into two, a process known as **mitosis**. During this process the DNA in the nucleus of this single cell replicates itself to form two nuclei. At the same time the cytoplasm divides and surrounds the two new nuclei, resulting in two cells, each enclosed by a membrane. The two new cells ('daughter cells' of the original) then divide to form four cells and so on.

Sometimes, however, this growth process goes wrong. For reasons not fully understood, part of the information carried in the DNA is altered, and an abnormal cell is formed. (This is known as **malignant transformation**.) This abnormal cell then divides as described above, eventually forming a cluster of abnormal cells which, if they survive, form a tumour.

Normal cells do not become malignant suddenly. There is a series of events which culminate in a cell growing out of control. These events take place long before the cancer becomes a problem. We know this because sometimes purely by chance some of the earlier changes can be seen. In the cells lining the small airways of the lung little areas of change can be detected by looking at the cells down a microscope. These changes are much commoner in heavy smokers who we know have a much greater chance of getting lung cancer. Such cells may divide faster, look abnormal and arrange themselves in a disorderly fashion.

TUMOURS

A tumour is a mass of tissue formed as the result of cells growing abnormally and excessively. These cells continue to grow indefinitely and without restraint. There are two types of tumour – **benign** or **malignant**. Broadly speaking, benign tumours are localised – that is, they do not spread from the part of the body in which they began. They often have a clear capsule – a rim of normal tissue which marks the limit of the tumour. They may be detected because as they grow they press on other important structures in the body such as blood vessels or the intestine. In the skin they cause blemishes which can easily be seen. A simple wart is a good example of a benign tumour. On the whole, benign tumours are easily removed by surgery and do not recur. It is only in rare cases – for example, if a benign tumour exists deep in a vital part of the brain where surgery is likely to cause serious damage – that this is impossible.

Malignant tumours (cancers), on the other hand, are virtually never surrounded by a capsule and they erode adjacent tissues and infiltrate other parts of the body, extending crablike projections in all directions. Indeed, when cancer was first described it was named after the Latin for a crab. With a few exceptions, the unequivocal feature of a malignant tumour is its ability to spread through the blood and lymph vessels and establish itself in other parts of the body. Doctors call this process **metastasis**.

Cancer cells

The components and structure of a cancer cell are essentially the same as those of a normal one. The most important difference is that cancer cells will continue to multiply, often outgrowing their blood supply and the space available. Most of them grow more rapidly than the normal cells from which they originated. Down the microscope cancer cells often look very different from each other and from their normal parents and often contain large, bizarre nuclei. One reason for this is that the cells grow so quickly they have no time to organise themselves, but just keep dividing.

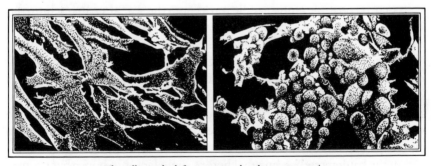

The cells on the left are normal – they stop growing
when they touch. The cells on the right are malignant – they are piling up
and have lost their normal growth restraint

The most dangerous feature of malignant tumours is their ability to spread to other parts of the body where they can generate new tumours. Scientists do not yet fully understand how this happens, but the fact that cells within the same tumour can look very different from each other suggests that cancer cells continually modify their behaviour during growth. It may be that during this process bits of DNA associated with a natural tendency to spread may become emphasised. The likelihood of tumours spreading, and the rate at which this occurs, varies from one type of tumour to another.

How Do Cancers Spread?

There are several ways in which cancer can spread. Cancer cells can pass into the lymph channels. These tiny pipes connect the lymph nodes in all parts of the body, ultimately draining into a large vein. The spread of the disease follows the natural routes of lymph drainage of the area. The bloodstream can also convey malignant fragments to distant parts. Cells can seed directly in body cavities such as the peritoneum within the abdomen or the lining around the lungs. Here cells break off the tumour and migrate in the fluid in which they bathe. The transplantation of tumour cells may be possible along needle tracks or in the scar after an operation. A cascade of events is involved between the shedding of a single cell by a primary tumour and the disease establishing itself in another part of the body.

Cancers do not spread in a haphazard or arbitrary way, and particular tumours have favoured sites. This is, to some degree, related to the routes of spread. Sarcomas (tumours arising from the body's structural tissues) often spread by showering cells into the bloodstream. Such cells get filtered by the small blood vessels in the lungs and so secondary tumours in the lungs are common. Prostate cancer seems to like growing in bone – often, the spine or pelvic bones. There is some factor in bone that encourages growth. Colon cancer often colonises the liver causing damage and eventually a reduction in the liver's ability to clear poisons from the blood.

But although we know which sites a particular type of tumour is likely to be found in, it is less easy to predict whether or not the disease will spread in any one person. One theory for this is that the body's own immune system may detect and engulf cancer cells as they travel. Another is that tumours that have begun in one part of the body may not necessarily be able to establish themselves in a different type of tissue. As yet, we do not know which factors make it possible for cancer cells to spread. An understanding of this process may be the key to curing cancer. We are already able to control the majority of solid, localised tumours with surgery or radiation. It is the cells that get away that can defeat us.

How Cancers Are Classified

Cancer can occur in any organ of the body. The behaviour pattern of cancer arising at different sites varies enormously. There are currently 206 classifiable sites at which tumours can arise and many of these can be broken down into further sub-types. This reflects the many different cells that go to make up the human body – many of which can evolve to grow out of control.

Tumours are classified by the site at which they originate. For example, a patient with breast cancer that has spread through the bloodstream to the liver is said to have metastatic breast cancer (i.e. breast cancer that has spread) and not a primary liver tumour.

This classification by likely site of origin often causes confusion to patients and families. Tumours are given a name reflecting the type of structure from which they have come. A **carcinoma**, for example, comes from cells lining body cavities. Such cells are found in the lung, colon, breast and in many other organs. Carcinomas are by far and away the commonest type. Tumours arising from the body's structural tissues – muscle, tendons, bones and cartilage – are called **sarcomas**. Those arising from the lymphatic system are called **lymphomas**; and cancers of the white blood cells in the bone marrow – **leukaemias**.

SYMPTOMS

Because there are many different types of cancer, there is no one way in which it first draws attention to itself. What happens first depends on the site and size of the tumour and on any spread of the disease as well as on any other medical problems a patient may have. For example, a small tumour on the vocal cord will rapidly create a small ulcer on the cord preventing its complete closure whilst speaking and leading to a hoarse voice. In this way a relatively tiny tumour produces the alarming symptom of persistent hoarseness driving the patient to the doctor rather quickly. Patients with lung cancer, on the other hand, often show no unusual symptoms until relatively late. The majority of such patients are smokers who are used to frequent coughing, shortness of breath and even occasional chest pains – all features of a growing tumour. By the time something really novel develops, such as the coughing up of a small amount of blood, the tumour has firmly established itself. Pain comes from the pressure on, or the destruction of, tissues containing nerve fibre endings. The centre of most organs contains no nerve endings and it is only when their outer lining is stretched that the patient notices something wrong.

Being aware of symptoms that may well be due to cancer is an important part of health education. An organ not functioning properly is one symptom, but there are many others that are much less specific. These include a feeling of tiredness, weakness, weight loss, fever, nausea and sweating at night. How these effects are produced is not always clear. The most likely explanation is that substances are released by tumour cells which trigger the symptoms indirectly. Of course, any of these may be caused by medical problems other than cancer. If any unusual symptom persists, you should see your doctor.

TYPES OF TREATMENT

Cancer treatment is often confusing even to many doctors not specialising in this field. The best treatment depends on a wide range of criteria – the age of the patient, whether preservation of fertility is important or possible, personal preference and even the distance to be travelled for therapy. The type of disease, its site and degree of spread are clearly vital factors in determining which treatment is best. We will look at all these in more detail, but here is a brief summary of the methods of treatment in current use.

Surgery is likely to be used to obtain a sample of tissue for diagnosis. In some cancers, where it is important that the bulk of disease is removed surgically, it can be an essential part of treatment. Nevertheless, it is a common misconception that in the last resort cancer can be cut out. Cancer cells cannot be distinguished accurately with the naked eye, so the surgeon cannot be completely certain all the tumour has been removed. Cells may sometimes be left behind and will soon fill the space made available by growing more rapidly.

Radiation has been used to treat cancer since its discovery over 100 years ago. Not all tumours are radio-sensitive, however.

Although chemotherapy (treatment with anti-cancer drugs) has been available for the latter half of this century, it is only in the past twenty-five years that it has seen widespread successful application. With an increasing number of type of compounds available, coupled with their decreased side effects and cost, some tumours have become curable. The vast majority of common tumours unfortunately remain relatively resistant to cure by chemotherapy. Moreover, certain drugs have serious long-term side effects: because of the later risk of cancer, for example, certain drugs are not used in the treatment of childhood cancers. As better agents and antidotes are uncovered, side effects such as hair loss and nausea are gradually being overcome.

Hormone therapy is suitable for a limited number of hormone-sensitive tumours – notably breast and prostatic cancer. If the tumour responds to hormonal adjustment it may control the spread of the disease for a number of years with little in the way of side effects for the patient. This is particularly likely in the elderly; younger patients tend to have more aggressive tumours which are not so responsive. Hormone treatment can usually be taken as simple tablets, making life easy.

There are no hard and fast rules in the treatment of cancer. Everybody is different, so it's not really surprising that when they become ill their needs will differ. The treatments available for cancer have become very sophisticated. The difficulty for the specialist is to know how best to combine them for an individual. In addition the situation must be continuously reassessed. Is the tumour responding to treatment? What are the side effects and are they likely to limit the dose of drugs or radiation given? If so, will this reduce the chance of cure? All these questions must be constantly reviewed to achieve the best results.

THE FUTURE

Sadly, anybody and everybody can develop cancer. There is no watertight avoidance strategy. There are some general principles suggested in the next chapter and it is sensible to follow these. Individuals who have a strong family history of cancer are more at risk, particularly with inherited cancers or those where there is a strong inherited trait (such as breast, colon and ovarian cancer). In these situations members of the family can be screened regularly. As further advances occur, it should be possible to detect malignancies at a very early stage without resorting to surgery.

Although statistics tell us that cancer is becoming more common, many cancers related to unhealthy habits (e.g. smoking-related lung cancers in men) are on the decline. What *has* altered is our ability to detect cancer at an earlier, treatable stage. Although tumours have been seen in the Egyptian mummies, they may not have always been diagnosed as cancer at the time. Cancer will be with us for many years to come. As we probe deeper and deeper into how cells grow and divide, we are getting down to the building blocks of life itself. It is here that the answer to cancer must lie. As we increase our understanding we will almost surely discover new methods of treating, and ultimately preventing, this important problem.

PREVENTING CANCER

'WHAT CAUSED IT, DOCTOR?'

This is one of the most common questions asked by patients who have cancer, and a tremendous amount of research has taken place over the last century to try to answer it. The first clear-cut observation was made by Percival Pott, a surgeon at St Bartholomew's Hospital in London in the eighteenth century. He noted that chimney sweeps were prone to get tumours of the skin surrounding the testicles. These poor boys were sent up chimneys at an early age and seldom got a wash. The various chemicals in soot accumulated in their groins and caused long-standing skin irritation, which eventually became malignant.

This was the first recognised example of an occupational cancer. Many others became apparent in this century: asbestos workers developing tumours in the lining around the lungs; uranium miners getting lung cancer; workers in the rubber industry using aniline dyes developing bladder cancer. Some cancers were shown to have a clear-cut single cause. Does all cancer have a specific cause or is it the inter-relationship between many different factors that leads to cancer?

The answer is not straightforward. Many factors can trigger off the disease, but it is very difficult to disentangle *which* factors are important in the development of an individual patient's cancer. To understand the complexity of the situation, the concept of probability must be introduced.

If you travel on an aeroplane, there is a small but definite risk that it will crash. Let's say that the aeroplane has four jet engines, like a Boeing 747 – the jumbo jet. The chances of one engine packing up are very small. But if, for example, a fire breaks out in the far right engine, the pilot can extinguish the fire successfully and fly on three engines. Now one of the other engines develops sudden vibration and fails. The pilot can still fly on two engines, although the journey becomes a bit more uncomfortable and manoeuvring difficult. Then suddenly, the third engine blows. The plane, whilst still able to hold its height, is unstable and very difficult to manoeuvre. A great strain is placed on that last engine. The chances of crashing now are much greater than they were at the start of the flight. If the last engine goes, then that's it.

The best way to think of cancer is as a series of engine failures in the growth control apparatus of the cell. Many of us may well be walking around with one or two cells already down the road to cancer, but no tumour has emerged. It needs several hits on the right targets within the DNA, inside the cell's nucleus, to cause cancer. If we stick with our aeroplane analogy, there are many factors that can cause 'engine failure'. But of course, the final straw is the last engine, and that may not always pack up.

Time is often said to be the greatest enemy. In the development of cancer, age is a major factor. Continuing our jumbo jet analogy, the chances of things going wrong increase with time as we fly across the Atlantic. Similarly, the chances of a cell going astray in our body increase as we travel on in our journey through life. There are certain exceptions to this. Certain childhood tumours – leukaemias, brain and kidney tumours – may occur even in newborn children. Testicular cancer peaks in men in their twenties and thirties, again suggesting that the events that led to them occurred early during adolescence or even before. But the vast majority of common tumours occur in the fifth and sixth decades of life and increase in incidence subsequently. This bears out the multi-hit theory; the fact that several events have to take place for most of these tumours.

Much as we would like to, we cannot stop time, and therefore the ageing process. What we *can* do is identify those factors in our lifestyle that may increase our cancer risk and do something about them.

INHERITED CANCER

We all have different faces, body sizes and shapes, intelligence, characters and fingerprints. Underneath what we can see, we each possess our own molecular sequences of DNA. On the whole, patients with cancer can be reassured that the disease is not hereditary and their children are not at greater risk from the disease but, for reasons that we do not fully understand, some of us may well be more susceptible to develop specific cancers than others.

There are certain very rare tumours which do behave in a classic genetic way. Retinoblastoma, a very unusual eye tumour in the retina at the back of the eye, behaves according to strict genetic rules. The genes are carried from father to son and from mother to daughter, resulting in a nearly 50 per cent chance of retinoblastomas in the offspring. Children of such families, which are fortunately very rare, are screened from an early age to look for eye tumours and the disease can now be cured by early surgery and radiotherapy.

Breast cancer is very common, with one in twelve women in Britain developing the disease. The incidence is almost one in two in certain families. Although the disease is not passed on by strict genetic rules, the tendency to develop it clearly runs in the family. Screening such families to pick up tumours early is of great value, and increases the chances of successful treatment. There are other examples of families where there is a much higher incidence of cancer than expected. Some of these families may have difficulty in repairing damage to the DNA caused by chemical and physical agents. Or their genes may be very sensitive to such agents. In either case, the risk of developing cancer is higher than normal.

Reducing your cancer risk

The vast majority of cancers are *not* hereditary and, even if a close relative has had the disease, you are at no greater risk of developing it.

Those rare cancers which *may* be hereditary include retinoblastoma, childhood kidney cancer and (in some cases) breast and ovarian cancer.

You can't choose your family, so the most positive step you can take is to be aware of any potential risk and look out for possible symptoms. If a close relative of yours has had one of these cancers, ask your doctor about screening programmes – that is, regular check-ups so that if you do develop symptoms they can be detected and treated at an early stage.

Early detection is an essential part of cancer prevention and all women, not just those with a family history of breast cancer, should regularly check their breasts for any lumps which might indicate a tumour (see illustration). Most breast lumps are completely harmless, but even those that are cancerous can often be treated succesfully.

F A C T S   A T   Y O U R   F I N G E R T I P S

- Most cancers are *not* hereditary.
- Make a list of your family, starting with your grandparents and including your father, mother, brothers, sisters, aunts, uncles and first cousins. Mark any that have had cancer and note its type. If more than two have had cancer, consult your doctor.
- If you think your family may be at risk of developing a rare familial cancer (e.g. retinoblastoma, childhood kidney cancer), ask your doctor about regular screening programmes.
- Regular breast self-examination (once a month) is essential for *all* women, as are check-ups by your GP or local Well Woman Clinic.
- Screening programmes are now available for ovarian cancer. Ask your doctor for details.

CHEMICAL CAUSES

The realisation that chemicals cause cancer came from the early observations of Percival Pott, followed by experimental work in the 1920s in London. A group of research workers at the Institute of Cancer Research were fascinated by the observation that coal tar extracts obtained from the Fulham gasworks could cause cancers of the skin in mice. They began to analyse the cancer-causing components of coal tar, and found that specific chemical structures were responsible. Such chemicals are called **carcinogens**.

Since the first discovery of carcinogens sixty years ago, many chemicals have now been shown to be damaging to cells, so increasing the chance of them becoming malignant. For some chemicals the risk is very high and easily spotted. A good example are the aniline dyes used to soften rubber for making tyres. It became very clear that people working in the manufacture of rubber materials stood a very high chance of getting bladder cancer. When aniline dyes were found to be responsible, far greater safety precautions were adopted and now there is no risk of factory workers ingesting the dye. Asbestos, which was used for pipe lagging and in shipbuilding, causes a very rare type of cancer of the membrane lining of the lung. This cancer, called mesothelioma, is extremely rare except in those who have been exposed to asbestos dust for long periods of time. Now rigid safety precautions are taken by those handling asbestos, including the use of special filter masks to prevent the fibres being breathed in. Asbestos is found in many older buildings, so when conversion work is done the area is sealed off by polythene sheeting. You may have noticed this together with the danger signs about asbestos.

There are many chemicals which are now known to cause cancer. Pollution from factories and the increased use of very potent chemicals in modern farming increases the chances of our exposure to them. But because we are usually exposed at only a low dose and for a short period of time the chances of getting cancer are relatively low. It is unlikely that pollution adds more than a fraction of a percentage to our overall cancer risk.

SMOKING

Compounds similar to coal tar were found in cigarette smoke. It is very surprising now to imagine that thirty years ago cigarettes were not recognised as a major cause of lung cancer. Look at any of the great old films of the 1940s and early 1950s. The Bogart movies such as *Casablanca* are perhaps the best examples. Nearly every character seems to be smoking at some stage. The film director used cigarette smoke creatively in moments of great poignancy. Smoking was freely permissible in all public places in the UK, even in hospitals, cinemas and London's Underground.

Things began to change when Richard Doll and his colleagues at Oxford began to survey patients with lung cancer and compare them with patients of similar age and sex who did not have the disease. They found that nearly all the lung cancer patients smoked heavily whilst very few of the control group did. This observation was contested fiercely by the tobacco companies and those who had a vested interest in the sale of tobacco. They suggested that there were many other factors responsible, such as a different lifestyle of smokers compared with non-smokers. There was evidence, for example, that smokers had a higher sugar intake than non-smokers.

Doll then went on to establish his now classic study on British doctors. Using a detailed questionnaire, followed up at regular intervals, he collected data on the change in smoking habits of many GPs. A comparison was made between those who had stopped smoking and those who had continued, and a clear pattern emerged. Those doctors who had stopped smoking considerably reduced their risk of getting lung cancer. In other words, even heavy smokers can redeem themselves if they stop in time.

The growing body of evidence linking cigarettes to lung cancer and subsequently to heart disease and chronic bronchitis, has finally led to a change in public opinion, with the government banning cigarette advertising on television and in many other situations. However, many sporting events still have large slogans suggesting either the association of cigarettes with health in physical sports, or with sexual prowess in others, such as motor racing. The tobacco lobby still continues. The chairman of Rothman's International recently stated, 'there is no evidence that ciga-

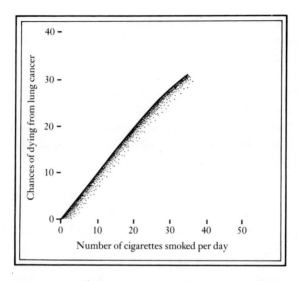

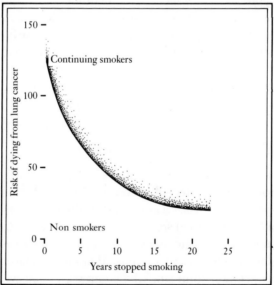

The risk of lung cancer increases steadily with the number of cigarettes smoked, and starts to decrease as soon as someone stops smoking

rettes cause lung cancer'. But gradually the tide of public opinion has turned and smokers are now being shunned more and more.

The realisation that breathing in the exhaled smoke of others – passive smoking – can also lead to a significant increase in the incidence of cancer, has resulted in public demand for smoke-free areas on transport, in leisure areas and in the work place. Courts can protect the right of an individual to choose whether to smoke or not. The evidence accumulating on passive smoking suggests that those that wish to continue to smoke should do so in the privacy of their, hopefully well-ventilated, room. A good analogy would be a passenger on a transatlantic flight wishing to switch off one of the engines to see what happened just for fun. The rest of the passengers would be compelled to take part in this dangerous experiment.

Of course, heavy smokers rationalise, rather like the tobacco industry. 'My grandfather smoked fifty cigarettes a day and lived until he was eighty', is a common reply from patients where attempts are being made to reduce their smoking. The opposite is sometimes used: 'My mother died of lung cancer at fifty and she never smoked a single cigarette in her life.' These statements, which are often exaggerated, show the failure to understand the statistical nature of the disease. Another argument is that you have to die from something anyway. This is true, but lung cancer does affect men and women in their fifties and sixties – well below the average age of death. It is also an unpleasant disease to have.

Reducing your cancer risk

Stopping smoking – or, better still, never starting – is the single biggest way of reducing your cancer risk. Of course it is difficult to stop completely. If you are a heavy smoker, then start by trying to cut down. Limit your cigarette consumption to specific times of the day. Change to a low-tar brand. Do not inhale the smoke. Use a longer filter and milder cigarette. Then make the big step: abandon smoking completely. You will be surprised how healthy you will feel a month or so later. Breathing will be easier, you will cough less and will feel fitter and more able to go about life. Many

F A C T S   A T   Y O U R   F I N G E R T I P S

Stop smoking now!

- One third of all cancer deaths are caused by smoking.
- Lung cancer causes 40 000 deaths a year in the UK – that's about 110 every day.
- If you smoke twenty cigarettes a day, you are forty times more likely to get lung cancer than a non-smoker.
- Your risk of developing other tumours – in your liver, gall bladder, bladder or pancreas – is also increased if you smoke.
- Your risk of developing cancer begins to fall as soon as you give up smoking.

If you really can't give up immediately:

- Cut down by only allowing yourself to smoke at certain times of the day.
- Change to a low-tar brand.
- Always use filter tips.
- Inhale less smoke.
- Ask your doctor about anti-smoking clinics and other ways of helping you to stop.

If you are a non-smoker:

- Campaign for a no smoking environment.
- Insist on a smoke-free work place.
- Make a fuss! If someone says, 'Do you mind if I smoke?' don't be afraid to say that you *do* mind.
- Discourage your children from smoking.

arguments against stopping smoking are put forward. O.K., so you may put on a little weight as you transfer nervous activity from cigarettes to food. You may start drinking a little more alcohol. This does not matter in the short term because these habits, too, can be curbed later once you have given up smoking. Find out about anti-smoking clinics locally. Your GP will be in the best position to advise. There are various aids that can be used including nicotine-containing chewing gum.

If you are a non-smoker, then campaign for a no smoking environment. This will reduce the risk of your getting cancer by passive smoking and also provide an atmosphere where smokers are shunned. How many times have you started coughing when a colleague has lit up a cigarette? Personal liberty is a grand-sounding title for the ability to poison your colleagues. Insist on a smoke-free work place. Recent changes in public transport laws are leading the way. The London Underground system has abolished smoking altogether, although this is probably related to a disastrous fire in 1987 rather than concern for the health of its customers. Airlines have started non-smoking flights, usually on short domestic routes so as not to affect international customers. There is nothing worse than being a non-smoker in a plane, sitting on the boundary between smoking and non-smoking areas. Support such measures.

Above all, discourage your children from smoking. This is the key to the future. The tobacco industry spends millions on advertising, whereas health education spends a paltry sum. The two are mutually conflicting. If we can dissuade teenagers from taking up smoking, the next generation will reap the benefits.

DIET

The diet we eat today is not the one our bodies were designed to take. The basic problem is that our diet has become highly refined, concentrated and of course, on occasions, delicious. Man evolved as a hunter, searching where he could for food, eating both plants and animals. If we could put Stone Age man in a time machine and send him for dinner at a fancy Paris restaurant, or to the local fast-food burger store, not only would he find the surroundings strange, but he would find the food almost inedible. Let's just take a look at the modern hamburger, the sort children clamour for when offered a meal out. It is usually served with chips, a cola drink or a milkshake.

The first problem is the fat content. As much as 70 per cent of the leanest-looking burger may in fact consist of animal fat. For many years now it has been recognised that the incidence of breast cancer follows closely the daily average fat consumption (see illustration below). Those countries where women have a high fat intake have a high level of the disease. Moreover, fat dramatically increases the calorie content – something to be avoided if you're trying to keep your weight down. Preservatives will be added to the meat to keep it fresh, as will a range of colourings and

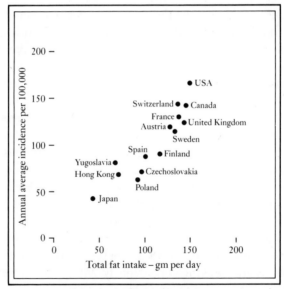

*In a study of 14 countries, the incidence of breast
cancer (number of cases per 100,000 women) was found to increase
in line with the average daily intake of fat*

unknown chemicals. The burger will be grilled, producing coal-tar-like compounds on its outside which can be carcinogenic. The bun itself will be white, made from the most refined flour, having very little fibre content. The chips will be coated in fat and may well have added chemicals to increase the crispness of their outer coat. The cola drink will contain the equivalent of ten sugar lumps. The milkshake will be made from full-fat milk and chemical flavourings, all potentially dangerous.

Having the odd meal out at a burger joint is not a bad thing once in a while, but a fast-food structured diet is asking for trouble. There is evidence that the sort of foods we eat can, in the long term, determine the incidence of cancer. Evidence for this comes from comparing the incidence of cancer in populations with radically different diets. In Africa, for example, the diet is mainly vegetarian with a high content of fibre; this results in the average African producing over a kilogram of stool daily, in contrast with the average Westerner who produces less than 300 grams. The incidence of colorectal cancer is high in the West, but almost non-existent in Africa. The reason for this is the reduced transit time in the intestine caused by the high bulk of African stool. The increased transit time in Westerners allows carcinogenic chemicals in our diet to sit in contact with the bowel wall. Another reason may well be the bacteria that inhabit the intestine. The rapid transit time may change the composition of organisms, some of which may not be able to produce the unpleasant carcinogens that we get in the West.

Furthermore, obesity will be a problem. This alone has an increased cancer risk in certain areas of the body. Obesity is, of course, a health hazard in many ways, other than increasing cancer risk. Heart disease, high blood pressure, arthritis, psychological disturbances and strokes are all increased in patients who are fat. It is not only grossly obese people who have these increased risks. If you go to any pub on a Sunday lunchtime, you will find a group of men with pot-bellies usually standing at the bar, many of whom are smoking continuously. Middle-age spread is induced by too much eating, partly caused by good home cooking and also too much drinking of high-calorie fluids, such as beer.

Reducing your cancer risk

It is not always easy to alter your lifestyle. If you are in a group which meets regularly before Sunday lunch to drink beer in the pub, there is a lot of peer pressure to continue to do so. Asking for a tonic water instead of a pint may

---

F A C T S   A T   Y O U R   F I N G E R T I P S

- Don't worry too much about preservatives in food – on the whole, they do more good than harm.
- If you are overweight – slim! As well as increasing your risk of certain types of cancer, being obese (that is, 40 per cent or more above the recommended weight for your height and build) can give rise to a number of other medical problems.
- Eat less fat
    - switch from hard cooking fat to oil
    - avoid fried food
    - use less butter or switch to a low-fat spread
    - use skimmed milk instead of full fat milk
    - use cottage cheese instead of solid cheese
- Eat less sugar
    - cut down on (or do without) sugar in tea and coffee
    - cut down on sweets and snacks
    - avoid fizzy drinks
- Increase the amount of fibre that you eat. Fibre occurs in bran cereals, brown bread, fruit.
- Make sure you get plenty of vitamins naturally
    - eat plenty of fruit
    - don't overcook vegetables (this prevents vitamins from being destroyed, and undercooked vegetables taste better, anyway)
- The occasional fast-food meal won't do you any harm – but don't let it become a habit!

---

well be met with derision. Again, there are vested interests at stake trying to stop you adopting a sensible, healthy lifestyle. The breweries and publicans make their money by selling beer and do not wish to portray beer-drinking as a cause of obesity.

Once you see through this ploy, it becomes easier to change things. Reducing weight is not as difficult as stopping smoking, mainly because you can still eat. The first thing to do is to review your behaviour patterns, go through the average day and look at what you are eating. Take breakfast: if you have a cooked breakfast, is it necessary? The standard British breakfast sold in hotels and on the railway is one of the most unhealthy starts imaginable. Whilst it is fun once in a while, to have such a meal every day is asking for trouble. Many people do not have a cooked breakfast as such, but eat a high calorie intake with fat in the form of butter, calories in the form of jams and marmalades. What kind of cereal are you taking? Is it made from highly purified grain, or does it contain fibre? These small changes over a long period of time can result in big differences in cancer risk. At lunchtime, do you have a cooked lunch or just a sandwich? Is it sausages and chips every day with all the problems of fast food? Or is it a more sensible meal with salad and fruit? In the evening is it more fast food or a balanced diet? What about snacks between meals, which are often very high in calories? A well-known advertisement for a chocolate-coated bar states that it will help you work, rest and play. The only health gain in this bar is the bank balance of the producer's shareholders. An occasional bar will do no harm but regular eating of chocolates, however delicious, can lead to obesity and all its problems. Unfortunately, it is difficult to be dogmatic about dietary advice. But there are some definite pointers which will help you foil cancer.

ALCOHOL

The association between alcohol and cancer is complex, for it seems to depend on the way in which alcohol is taken as well as on the amount. In France, large quantities of wine are consumed regularly from an early age.

There is good evidence that cancer of the mouth and oesophagus (the tube connecting the mouth to the stomach) are associated with heavy wine consumption. Alcohol in any form in excess causes serious liver damage. Liver cells die and are replaced by defective cells which causes fibrosis of the liver. This is called cirrhosis. Alcoholic cirrhosis causes a high incidence of liver cancer in later life. The type of liver cancer it produces is often widespread in the liver and not amenable to most treatments. Small amounts of alcohol are not dangerous, but excess drinking over a period of time will result in increased cancer incidence. Perhaps more important, of course, are the problems of addiction with inability to carry on an effective job and the breakdown of family life that chronic alcoholism can produce. There is a slippery slope about alcohol intake. Casual drinking can lead to heavy bouts of drinking and subsequently addictive behaviour patterns, such as drinking alone or early in the morning.

Reducing your cancer risk

The recommended level of 'safe' drinking is no more than 21 units a week for men and no more than 14 units a week for women. (A unit is equivalent to ½ pint of beer or cider, or 1 single measure of spirits, or 1 glass of wine.) Count up how many units you drink in an average week – you may get a nasty shock!

F A C T S   A T   Y O U R   F I N G E R T I P S

- Excess alcohol causes 3 per cent of all cancers.
- Limit your alcohol intake: no more than 21 units a week for men and no more than 14 for women.
- Take low-alcohol or non-alcoholic drinks.
- Try not to drink every day.
- Do not drink regularly to relieve stress.
- Do not feel obliged to drink just because other people are.
- Seek help if you cannot stop drinking.

If you think you may be drinking too much, try to cut down. Drink low-alcohol or non-alcoholic drinks instead, and try to go for two or three days without drinking any alcohol at all. In the pub or at a party, space out your alcoholic drinks – have a glass of wine and then a mineral water or a fruit juice. Don't drink regularly to relieve stress. And above all, don't feel obliged to drink just because other people are.

PHYSICAL AGENTS

We are all exposed to the physical agents of our environment daily. Heat, light, X-rays, gamma rays are all unavoidable in the world in which we live. Under certain conditions, these can cause DNA damage in cells and result in growth-control abnormalities.

SUNSHINE

Have you ever wondered why the piers dotted around Britain's coasts are so run down? Many are closed and those that are open are shadows of their former selves. This sad decline reflects the change in holiday pattern for most Britons. The availability of modern jet travel, coupled with development of cheap tourist hotels along the Mediterranean coast, has led many families to take their summer holiday abroad. Even on the hottest summer day, the British sunshine is relatively timid compared to that of the Mediterranean or other far-away places.

It has been known for some time that ultra-violet radiation from the sun can cause cancer of the skin, predominantly in the exposed areas of the face and hands, and especially in fair-skinned people. People who live in hot climates tend to have darker skin. The pigment in the skin absorbs the ultra-violet light, preventing too much damage. Thus, the skin cancer incidence amongst the Aborigines of Australia is very low, but amongst the migrants from Europe is the highest in the world. Although we think of sunbathing as a pleasant and healthy pursuit, the 'lobster look' achieved by so many on their Mediterranean holiday can actually increase the chances of getting certain types of skin cancer at a later date. As well as appearing pretty unpleasant, the lobster look has hidden dangers. The amount of ultra-violet light received by certain cells in the skin can result in serious damage to DNA. This in turn can lead to the subsequent development of cancers. Many skin cancers are easy to treat by surgery or radiotherapy. But there is one type that can spread and kill – the melanoma. Recent evidence has shown that melanoma incidence has increased rapidly in communities where sun is not a normal feature in their daily life, but where a large number go for sun exposure on their holidays.

Reducing your cancer risk

The lobster look is easy to avoid. The first step is not to expose large parts of the body immediately. Do it slowly. You can get a perfectly reasonable tan over a two-week period without lying on the beach for the whole of the first day. The second step is to use barrier creams which protect the skin

---

FACTS AT YOUR FINGERTIPS

- Only stay in the sun for a short period to begin with.
- Use a sunscreen, starting with a total block (factor 15) and reducing gradually to factor 7 as your tan builds up.
- Don't be fooled into thinking that just because there's a cool breeze from the sea you aren't likely to get sunburnt. You are – it's just that because the air temperature is cooler, you won't notice until it's too late.
- Avoid using sunbeds at home. Only use them when supervised at a health centre. Do not go for a rapid tan but allow your skin to darken over a period of several weeks. If you are naturally pale, be especially careful to limit exposure to 15 minutes a day to start with.

---

against the harmful elements of the sun's rays. These creams are now widely available and are very reasonably priced. The use of such creams will considerably reduce your risk of getting sunstroke and, in some cases, enhance your sun tan. Cheap alcohol in many resorts often results in holidaymakers over-indulging at lunchtime and then lying on the beach sleeping for the rest of the afternoon. This is extremely dangerous, both in the short term, because of sunstroke, and in the longer term because of the danger of melanoma. Similar problems may arise with certain artificial tanning devices.

RADIATION

Far more serious, as it remains unseen and in some cases not fully understood, is the effect of radiation. When Wilhelm Konrad Roentgen discovered X-rays in 1895 and Madame Curie isolated radium in the following year, the radiation age had dawned. It took some four years before the real power of radiation became apparent. The early workers in this area soon developed serious problems. Anaemia and a lowering of their white blood count was noted, making them susceptible to infections and later development of a variety of cancers. During the First World War, large armies of workers sat in huge aircraft hangars painting dials with luminous paint for the control panels of ships and planes. The luminous paint contained small amounts of radium which over the years impregnated the workers' skin. To get a fine point on the brushes necessary for the intricate work they would lick the brush, swallowing small amounts of radium. They too developed anaemia because of failure of the blood-forming cells, and also hideous mouth cancers which were incurable. It is paradoxical that the discovery of radium led to so many cancers as well as providing a cure. The uranium miners of South Africa, who live and work in an atmosphere laden with radon gas, suffer from a much higher incidence of lung cancer than ordinary coal miners. Again, this is due to radioactivity.

But the most dramatic introduction to the radiation age was the dropping of Trinity – the code name for the first atomic bomb dropped on

Hiroshima, followed shortly by another on Nagasaki. At first, the true power of the bomb was not realised, although the immediate devastation halted the Second World War and held the world in awe. Out of the rubble of Hiroshima and Nagasaki, a more terrible problem emerged. Areas of countryside remained radioactive for long periods of time. Men, women and children rebuilt the cities whilst the background radiation continued to destroy targets in their DNA. The measurement of radiation was very crude in the post-war era. Even so, current estimates suggest that exposure to relatively small amounts of radiation results in a much higher incidence of certain cancers. Initially, tumours occurred in the cells of the blood-forming system – leukaemias, with the common cancers such as those of lung, breast and colon following.

We are familiar with the evocative photographs of the British and French tests of atom bombs in the early 1950s, with the conscripted soldiers lined up against the mushroom cloud of fall-out. Rather like cigarette smoking, it is now difficult to understand why people did not take more precautions. It would be unthinkable today to carry out such tests in the open and to expose even volunteers to the types of doses these men were receiving.

The disaster at Chernobyl in the USSR in 1986 will give us considerable information about the long-term effects of radiation. The tragedy will be closely monitored, with over 30 000 people undergoing annual checks to compare the dose they received and the subsequent development of various cancers. Sadly, there appears to be no threshold of safe radiation. This means we must strive for the minimal possible exposure. But the risks are all relative.

Reducing your cancer risk

We live in the radiation age. We use X-rays for diagnosis and therapy, we produce electricity in nuclear power stations, and we use atomic bombs for political reasons to hold the balance of power between various countries. In addition, we are part of a universe where radiation is very much part of life. What can we do to minimise our exposure? The evidence that people living next door to a nuclear power plant or a hospital radiation therapy department have a higher risk of developing cancer is very weak. Recent surveys have shown a small increase in cancer risk in children living in West Cumbria near the Sellafield nuclear processing plant. But many factors are involved and the relationship of radiation to the higher incidence of leukaemia found here is very complicated. We must all play our part in campaigning to keep our environment safe. There are some types of radiation we can do very little about – for example, cosmic rays from the sun or the emissions from radon in certain building materials. But thanks to the setting-up of rigorous safety procedures, there is little risk of cancer from radiation used in the workplace. People working in X-ray departments, or in factories where X-rays are used, do not have a higher incidence of cancer.

The casual use of X-rays for shoe fitting has stopped, but still too many X-rays are performed unnecessarily in our hospitals. You have a personal responsibility for your health, and if an X-ray is requested by your doctor, you are quite entitled to ask how it will help in your diagnosis and treatment. One of the biggest bugbears of medicine is the frequent repetition of blood tests and X-rays by junior doctors to avoid any criticism that they have left out important tests.

A major dilemma has crept in with mammography in breast cancer screening. Mammograms (X-rays of the breast) are a very good way of telling if a patient has a small lump that may be malignant. Mammographic screening is about to be introduced in the UK, but there are many opponents to it. The opponents say that the X-rays used for the mammogram will in fact increase the risk of breast cancer. Unfortunately, we have no solid information either way. The individual X-ray dose accumulated over a large number of years may well be significant. There appears to be no lower threshold for cancer induction by radiation. This means that even trivial amounts of radiation may be important. Unborn babies and children are more susceptible as their tissues are more easily damaged. It has been shown that women who have had X-rays during pregnancy have a higher risk of producing abnormal babies. The most sensitive period is the first three months. Therefore, if you think you may be pregnant, tell your doctor before he sends you off for X-rays. Some X-ray investigations involve a much bigger dose of radiation than others. X-rays performed at the dentist, for example, use almost trivial amounts of radiation, whereas those to examine the kidneys may require a large amount. The best advice if you are pregnant is to keep asking the doctors and radiographers about the need for the investigation and whether it can be delayed until the pregnancy is completed. Certain types of investigation can even cause young children who are being breast-fed (see case history) to become radioactive.

F A C T S A T Y O U R F I N G E R T I P S

- Avoid unnecessary X-ray examinations – this is particularly important for pregnant women.
- Observe safety regulations meticulously.
- Campaign for a safer environment.

BIOLOGICAL FACTORS

Is cancer infectious? This is another common question in the clinic. The answer to nearly every patient is 'No'. But there are cancers in animals which are caused by viruses, and there are some human tumours which are either directly caused by, or related to, viral infection.

Viruses

In 1910 Peyton Rous, working in a laboratory in New York City, was puzzled by an observation he made. A farmer friend told him that some of his chickens developed curious sarcomas, tumours under the skin around the thigh. He did an experiment which showed that a cell-free extract of the tumour could actually cause tumours in other chickens. He had discovered the virus that bears his name, the Rous sarcoma virus (RSV). There are many similar viruses which cause tumours in hamsters, rats, mice, cats and even chimpanzees.

By 1970 a lot of information had been gathered about these viruses, but none had been found directly to infect humans. Then, a very puzzling observation was made. Along the coast of southern Japan, there are many fishing communities. The communities are very close-knit as access to many of the villages is difficult, some being accessible only by boat. In the local hospital it was noted that many villagers were getting a curious tumour of the lymph glands, called a T-cell lymphoma. Sometimes they had a form of leukaemia; instead of the lymph nodes being enlarged, the abnormal cells from the lymph nodes burst out into the circulation and could be seen in the blood under the microscope. T-cell lymphoma is incredibly rare in most parts of the world, but relatively common in fishing villages of southern Japan. Blood from these patients was collected and found to cross-react to a virus similar to Rous sarcoma virus. Subsequently a virus was isolated from material collected from one of the patients. The virus was called Human T-cell Lymphoma Virus 1, or HTLV1. Although a very rare cause of human cancer, the virus was to become enshrined in the history of medicine. It subsequently led to the discovery of its close relative HTLV3, now called HIV, the Human Immunodeficiency Virus and cause of AIDS. The viruses are very similar in structure, although HTLV1 is not spread by the same routes. So far, it is the only virus of its type that has been directly associated with human cancer.

HIV, the virus which causes AIDS, has now become the most prominent of the viruses transmitted by sex. Although AIDS patients develop cancer (often a very rare type of skin tumour called Kaposi's sarcoma), the reason the disease is so lethal is that the immune system is essentially wiped out. This leads to infections going out of control, especially in the lungs. The virus probably does not cause the cancer directly but rather by removing the immune system's ability to deal with wayward cells when they arise.

It has been known for some time that communities where promiscuity is low have a lower incidence of cervical cancer. Furthermore, such tumours often contain small viruses related to those that cause simple warts – the human papilloma virus. Recent observations have implicated a specific type of papilloma virus – type 16 – in the majority of cancers of the cervix. Clearly it is not the *only* cause of the disease but it appears to be a major factor.

Dennis Burkitt, a British surgeon working in Uganda, was curious about a very unusual lymphoma which now bears his name. He noted it in children of various parts of Africa, such as Uganda – usually in the areas in which malaria was rife. Although often presenting itself in an advanced stage, with horrible lesions around the mouth and at the back of the eye, the disease could often be treated by very simple chemotherapy. In the late 1960s, a virus was discovered growing out of Burkitt's lymphoma tissue. This was called the Epstein-Barr virus. Quite by chance, Epstein-Barr virus was also found to be the cause of glandular fever, a very common disease in Britain. Glandular fever is not a cancer, although lymphocytes are stimulated to cause swelling in the throat and in the neck lymph nodes. Burkitt's lymphoma, however, is lethal unless treated. But there is a paradox: glandular fever is common in this country and in America, and yet the incidence of Burkitt's lymphoma is extremely low. Even to this day, the paradox has not been resolved. The most likely scenario is that the Epstein-Barr virus is just one of several factors which lead to Burkitt's lymphoma. Chronic malaria infection in the areas of the world where Burkitt's lymphoma is found can stimulate the immune system. The number of white blood cells increases dramatically so that there are many more target cells for the Epstein-Barr virus to hit. Although the immune system is stimulated by the malaria parasite, it may well not be so effective at controlling the regeneration of abnormal cells. This may make lymphocytes infected with Epstein-Barr virus grow in a more uncontrolled way, leading to the lymphoma.

Another common viral disease in the Third World that is definitely associated with a specific cancer type is hepatitis B. This can be spread by a variety of routes: eating infected shellfish, the infusion of contaminated blood, sexual intercourse and, on some occasions, by direct contact. It causes inflammation of the liver, hence the name hepatitis. Although the lives of some patients may be threatened by declining liver function with jaundice, most patients make a full recovery. About five per cent of patients in those countries where malnutrition is rife go on to develop chronic hepatitis after many years. It is under these conditions that cancer of the liver (**hepatoma**) seems to arise. The hepatitis virus is incorporated in the malignant cells, suggesting that it may play a part in causing the cancer. It may well be disrupting those genes responsible for normal growth control, as well as stimulating the abnormal growth of cells in certain areas of the liver.

Reducing your cancer risk

In the vast majority of cancers, there is no evidence to suggest that viruses are responsible. Generally speaking, cancer is not 'catching'. Where viruses have been implicated in the development of cancers (e.g. in Burkitt's lymphoma, and cancer of the liver following hepatitis), other factors such as malaria or malnutrition have played an important part.

The exception to this is cancers arising from sexually transmitted viruses. There are several links between sex and cancer. Nuns, for example, have a very low incidence of cervical cancer. Almost certainly, their lack of sexual partners reduces the risk of infection by viruses or other agents that may cause changes in the lining of the neck of the uterus. That is not to say, of course, that women who have many sexual partners will necessarily get cervical cancer, but just that the probability is increased. Prostitutes, who for many years have multiple partners, are at greatest risk, not only from AIDS but from cervical cancer. There is increasing evidence associating the disease with various wart viruses, although the relationship is complex. The best advice is to try and keep the number of sexual contacts to a minimum and to use barrier contraception which protects against direct contact with viruses.

The same advice applies to avoiding AIDS. Casual sex without condom usage is fraught with hazards and should be avoided. The most dangerous scenarios are in holiday areas where prostitutes may well have bi-sexual men on their list of customers. In some under-developed areas, screening for viral infection may not be possible and the risk is increased. The best advice one can give is to avoid casual sex completely.

Cancer of the penis is relatively rare now. It usually occurs in elderly men and is often associated with poor hygiene. It is declining rapidly because of the increased awareness of the importance of hygiene generally and obviously the increased facilities for washing. There is some evidence for linkage of this tumour with cancer of the cervix, in that the same virus types appear to be involved in triggering both diseases. Attention to personal hygiene, and using a condom during casual sex, are probably the two best measures to try and reduce the already low incidence further.

FACTS AT YOUR FINGERTIPS

- When visiting certain countries, vaccination against hepatitis is recommended. Ask your doctor for details.
- Avoid casual sex.
- Use a condom to reduce the risk of infection.
- Keep the number of sexual contacts to a minimum.
- See your doctor if you have any persistent discharge.
- Women who are, or who have been, sexually active should be screened for cervical cancer every three years.

HORMONAL FACTORS

Hormones are the chemical controllers of the body. They are released by the glandular structures of the body as signals to other organs to implement change. There are many different hormones, some of which have a very profound influence on the way cells grow in different tissues. Sex hormones, for example, control the growth and development of breasts and uterus in women, and testes in men. Cyclical release of the appropriate sex hormones in women results in the menstrual cycle: the shedding of the lining of the uterus at monthly intervals. Individuals have their own hormonal make-up. For many years it has been realised that certain hormonal patterns may be associated with a higher or lower incidence of cancer, most usually of the breast or uterus. The age of a woman when she had her first period, the number of pregnancies and her age at the time, whether or not she breast-fed her children, and the age at which she reached the menopause all affect hormone levels on the normal breast and thus the likelihood of cancer in this area.

There is considerable controversy as to the cancer risk involved in manipulating the hormonal systems of the body. Hormonal manipulation has been used for many years, either for birth control (the contraceptive pill) or to prevent bone destruction after the menopause in women (replacement therapy). Certain types of contraceptive pill, containing a high level of oestrogen, have been associated with a higher than normal incidence of cancer in the breast and uterus, whilst those with a low dose may well have a protective effect.

It is clear that subtle changes in our hormonal make-up can cause long-term and unfavourable changes in various structures. As we learn more about the various factors that control growth in many tissues, we may become aware of how manipulations in the hormonal system can affect these and change the pattern of cancer incidence.

F A C T S   A T   Y O U R   F I N G E R T I P S

- If you are taking oral contraceptives, make sure they are of the low oestrogen type. If you are not sure see your doctor.
- If you have taken the pill for many years, consider alternative forms of contraception.
- If your doctor recommends hormonal replacement treatment after the menopause, make sure you try to stop it after one or two years.
- Take part in the various screening programmes offered for breast and gynaecological cancers.

Taking Responsibility For Your Own Health

Many of our recommendations will reduce your chances of getting other diseases as well: of the heart, lungs, gallstones, kidney stones and the many unpleasant ailments related to the behaviour patterns of modern society. There has to be an element of singlemindedness about your approach. There is no way a heavy smoker will succeed in giving up smoking without tremendous willpower and drive. Similarly, if you are overweight, it is difficult to slim rapidly and not regain weight. But it is by no means impossible.

Taking a reasonable amount of exercise is also important. The evidence that lack of exercise is directly related to the risk of getting cancer is small. However, exercise is part of a healthy lifestyle that will reduce the risks of cancer. There is no need to get carried away. Many joggers ostentatiously running round in the latest jogging gear may be hammering their bodies in a dangerous way. Walking to work, using the stairs instead of the lift, going for a walk instead of lying on the beach all day on holiday – these are all ways of increasing exercise in moderation. They will all help you avoid the sedentary lifestyle which many of us lead.

There are some very easy examinations which you can (and should) carry out regularly yourself as a means of detecting symptoms early – for breast cancer in women and testicular cancer in men (see pages 46–7 and 49).

There are a few diseases for which screening programmes can be effective. The one that is clear-cut is cancer of the cervix. Here, we screen not for the tumour itself, but for the pre-malignant state in the lining of the neck of the uterus. Breast cancer screening is more controversial: some people feel that every woman should be screened from the age of thirty-five onwards, whilst others believe that the screening programme X-rays could actually result in an increased cancer risk. The whole area is shrouded with politics. No government wants to be seen to be standing in the way of promoting better health. But the cost of screening is enormous and the resources could be spent more productively in other areas to improve the health of the nation.

The best place for co-ordinating health screening is the general practitioner's surgery. We are very privileged in Britain to have such an excellent system of primary care. The GP is the best person to provide advice about screening, and can, in fact, organise most of it.

If after reading this you feel that there are aspects of your lifestyle that could be improved, but are not sure how to go about it, then consult your GP. If you are a heavy smoker, your doctor may put you in touch with local anti-smoking groups. If you are overweight, he or she will help by suggesting various diets and also by checking for other diseases associated with obesity such as high blood pressure. Use your GP as a counsellor. Any doctor would rather take your blood pressure today than see you in ten years' time in the middle of the night after you've had a stroke.

CANCER SCREENING

We know that people who have small tumours are less likely to have metastases and therefore respond better to treatment. It would therefore seem logical that detecting tumours early would give better results. Unfortunately, this does not always follow. Some very small tumours can be extremely aggressive, spreading widely before they can be detected by any known test. Furthermore, for every person found to have cancer, many more will have suspicious abnormalities on the screening test that will require further investigation. This greatly adds to the cost of screening and, of course, to the level of anxiety of those taking part.

Cervical cancer

By taking a small sample of cells from the cervix using a wooden spatula and smearing these cells onto a glass slide, changes in pattern can suggest the subsequent development of cancer. This allows appropriate and very simple treatment to take place long before a tumour appears. For this reason, cervical smears are a very effective screening method. Current recommendations suggest that they should be done every three years from the age of 25–40. They are performed by GPs, gynaecology, antenatal and family planning clinics. There is little controversy about their effectiveness.

Breast cancer

In 1988 the Department of Health started to plan for a national breast cancer screening programme. This was based on data from large studies in New York and Stockholm and a pilot study in Britain of the use of special X-rays of the breast (mammograms) and clinical examination in large groups of women. The whole area is filled with controversy.

Although the New York data clearly show an advantage for screening, the Stockholm data are not so clear. In the studies the specialists involved in reading X-rays and performing the clinical examinations become very experienced and adept at picking up abnormalities that may be missed when the techniques are adapted to the fast turnover necessary for community screening. Furthermore, although the lesions picked up on screening are small, this does not necessarily mean that such patients will actually do better. If spread has already occurred when the diagnosis is made, then early detection is not necessarily of value. It could be that rapidly growing and spreading tumours may be picked up more readily by screening. A further problem is how often to do mammograms. The current recommendation is every three years. Mammograms involve the use of X-rays which may themselves induce cancer. There is a risk with the screening procedure, unlike that of cervical screening.

A simpler and cheaper way of screening is for women to examine their own breasts for lumps on a regular basis, every month (see illustration).

For political reasons the current government is insisting that the breast cancer programme goes ahead. It looks good for politicians to say they were involved at the inception of something that will promote good health. But a lot of women may well have unnecessary surgery for lumps that turn out not to be malignant. This could create a lot of avoidable anxiety. It would seem wiser to wait until more data are available before starting on a nationwide programme. The money could be better spent on anti-smoking advertisements for the time being.

BREAST SELF-EXAMINATION

Stand with your arms hanging loosely by your sides and look at **1** your breasts in the mirror. Go through this checklist:

Is there:
- any change in the size, shape or colour of your breasts?
- any change in the nipples?
- any bleeding or discharge from the nipples?
- any unusual puckering or dimpling on the breast or nipple?
- any vein standing out in a way that's not usual for you?

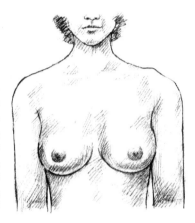

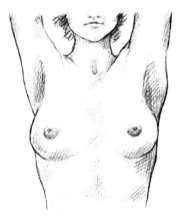

2 Now raise your arms above your head. Turn from side to side to see your breasts from different angles. Go through the checklist again.

Put your hands on your hips and press. Go through the checklist again.

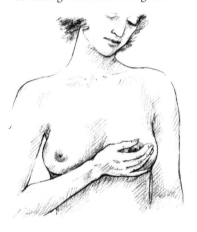

Squeeze each nipple gently to see if there's any bleeding or discharge. **3**

Lie down on your bed with your head on a pillow. Put a folded **4** towel under the shoulder blade of the side you are examining – this helps to flatten the breast tissue and makes it easier to examine.

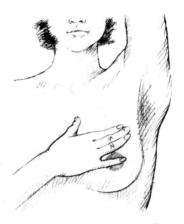

Use your left hand to examine your right breast and vice versa. Put the hand you're not using on the pillow under your head.

As you examine your breast, keep the fingers of the hand together. Use the flat of the fingers, not the tips.

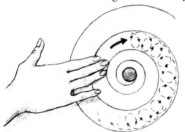

5 Trace a continuous spiral around the breast, moving your fingers in small circles and using firm pressure. Start by feeling around the nipple and then work outwards until you have felt every part of your breast. A ridge of firm tissue in a half-moon shape under the breast is quite normal: this helps to support your breast.

Bring the arm resting on the pillow down by your side. Using your left **6** hand to examine the right-hand side of your body, feel the part of your breast that goes up as far as the collarbone. Then feel the part that goes into the armpit. With the flat of the fingers again, feel for any lumps. Feel right up into the hollow of the armpit and work your way back towards your breast.

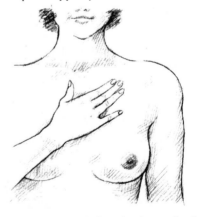

Now change sides and examine the other breast in exactly the same way with your other hand.

If you do find something unusual in one breast, always check the other breast for the same thing – it may just be the way your breasts are made.

Colon cancer

Although colon cancer is common, it often takes time for gastrointestinal symptoms, i.e. diarrhoea, abdominal pain and so on, to become apparent, by which time the disease is established. Such tumours eventually break through the lining of the colon and are directly exposed to the contents of the bowel. Here, they may bleed, producing a tiny trickle of blood. This goes unnoticed, until a moderately large blood vessel is eroded. There are chemical tests available to detect even traces of blood in the stool. An innovative approach has been to coat a detector for small amounts of blood onto toilet paper. If this changes colour, the patient is then asked to go and see their doctor. In the United States, the American Cancer Society is much more aggressive in its recommendations for screening for colorectal cancer. It recommends annual check-ups, including examination of the lower part of the colon, for everyone over the age of fifty-five. The evidence that this reduces the mortality from colorectal cancer remains to be seen.

Lung cancer

Until 1970, tuberculosis was fairly widespread in the UK. Chest X-rays were performed regularly to look for the disease. TB is now rarer and readily treatable but lung cancer has been increasing. Despite several studies with repeated chest X-rays to screen for lung cancer, no benefit has been found and although new patients are picked up by screening, there is no evidence that they respond better to existing therapy than those picked up when symptoms develop.

Testicular cancer

Although relatively rare, this type of cancer is easily treatable. It occurs mainly in young men. Regular self-examination (see illustration) will enable it to be detected at an early stage. See your doctor if you think there is an abnormality.

TESTICULAR SELF-EXAMINATION

1 You should examine your testicles regularly – say, once a month. It's easier to do this after a warm bath or shower, when the scrotal skin is relaxed. If you do notice anything unusual, make an appointment to see your doctor straightaway. It won't necessarily be cancer, but it's best to put your mind at rest.

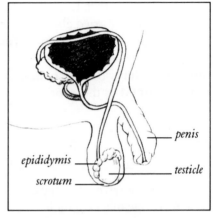

penis

epididymis

testicle

scrotum

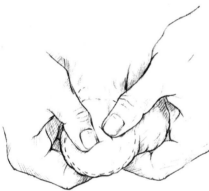

2 Hold your scrotum in the palms of your hands. This allows you to use the thumb and fingers of both hands to examine your testicles.

Note their size and weight. It's normal for one testicle to be larger than the other, but they should be roughly the same weight.

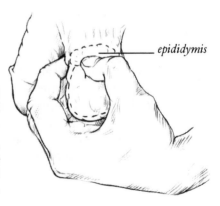

epididymis

3 Feel each testicle individually. You should be able to feel a soft tube at the top and back of the testicle. This is the epididymis, which carries and stores sperm and should not be confused with an abnormal lump.

Check each testicle for any lumps, swellings, slight enlargement or change in firmness. Normally, testicles should be smooth without any lumps.

There are several other experimental screening programmes for different tumour types. Rather than worry about whether to take part, the best advice is to take a high level of personal responsibility for your own health care. If you are worried about cancer, go and see your GP. He is the best person to advise about screening. The best indicator that something is seriously wrong, whether it be cancer or some other disease, is time. If a symptom persists for two weeks or more, medical advice should be sought. This is what your GP is there for.

C A N C E R   C H E C K L I S T

- A lump anywhere in the body.
- A change in a skin mole.
- A sore that doesn't heal.
- Any unusual bleeding in urine or stool, or in any discharge.
- Persistent diarrhoea or constipation.
- Persistent cough or hoarseness.
- Unexplained weight loss.

If you experience any of these, consult your doctor.

CONCLUSION

The probability of getting cancer is high with the disease affecting one in four of us. But we can tip the odds in our favour by adopting a sensible lifestyle. In doing so our level of health generally will improve and the chance of living to old age increases. Although there will be improvements over the next two decades, some of the most common cancers are likely to remain difficult to treat until well into the next century. More effort spent on prevention could pay big dividends.

Are You at Risk?

One in three of us will get cancer. We have outlined some of the ways we can avoid it. How does your lifestyle measure up? Complete the following questions and add up your marks.

	SCORE
Do you now smoke –	
nothing	0
less than 10 cigarettes/day	5
10–20 cigarettes/day	20
more than 20 cigarettes/day	30
an occasional cigar/pipe	4
Five years ago did you smoke –	
nothing	0
less than 10 cigarettes/day	3
10–20 cigarettes/day	12
more than 20 cigarettes/day	16
an occasional cigar/pipe	2

Is there a heavy smoker in your house or the room in which you work –

yes	2
no	0

Take your height in metres and multiply it by itself. Take your weight in kilograms and divide it by this number. Is your score –

MEN	WOMEN	
20–25	19–24	0
26–27	25–26	6
more than 27	more than 26	10

Do you eat fast food, e.g. hamburgers, hot dogs, fish and chips –

more than once weekly	3
less than once weekly	2
rarely	1

Do you eat meat –
    twice daily   2
    once daily   1
    occasionally/never   0

Do you eat a high fibre cereal for breakfast –
    every day   0
    three times weekly   1
    rarely   3

You are being taken out for dinner in your favourite restaurant. Which of the following items on the menu would you prefer –

    vegetable soup   0
    prawn cocktail   1

    brown bread   0
    white bread   1

    avocado vinaigrette   0
    deep-fried mushrooms   1

    chicken salad   0
    steak and chips   1

    chips   1
    baked potato   0

    gooseberry pie and cream   1
    fresh fruit salad   0

    black forest gateau   2
    cream caramel   0

Do you go abroad for holidays to a warmer climate –
    yes   1
    no   0

Do you use a barrier sun cream at least at the start of the holiday –

yes	0
no	1

Does your skin go bright red for several days before a tan develops –

yes	3
no	0

Does your job involve strenuous physical labour –

yes	0
no	1

Do you exercise or perform a physical sport at least once a week –

yes	0
no	2

Do you walk at least one mile on an average day –

yes	0
no	2

If you are a woman, do you take a contraceptive pill –

yes	1
no	0

How many sexual partners have you had –

none	0
1–5	1
5–10	2
more than 10	3

If you have sexual relationships, do you use a barrier contraceptive method, e.g. condom or cap –

yes	0
no	1

How many first degree relatives (i.e. father, mother, brother, sister) have had cancer –

none	0
1	1
2	2
more than 2	5

How much alcohol do you drink per week (one unit is one gin, whisky etc. or one half-pint of beer, lager or cider) –

none	0
1–14	2
14–30	4
more than 30	6

Well, how did you get on? If you have been honest, then you can get an impression of your relative cancer risk. For most things, including smoking, it is not too late to change.

SCORE

80–100 Very high cancer risk. You smoke heavily and are likely to be overweight. It's not just cancer that will kill you. Now is the time to change. See your doctor soon.

60–80 You have a high chance of getting cancer. You must cut down on smoking. Look at the rest of your lifestyle.

40–60 Watch it. Take the advice offered and review how you live.

20–40 Not bad. But be careful and follow the advice.

0–20 Low cancer risk. Keep going. There's no guarantee you won't get the disease, but you're doing all you can to avoid it.

DIAGNOSIS

J ust as no two individuals are alike, no two cancers are exactly the same. There are many symptoms which might indicate cancer, and different symptoms cause different degrees of alarm in patients and their families. For example, the coughing up of a small amount of blood, a gnawing chest pain, or persistent profound diarrhoea rapidly send patients to see their doctor. However, a slight shortness of breath, a general feeling of fatigue and loss of appetite may be ascribed to some temporary illness and shrugged off. How is the diagnosis of cancer made?

As we have explained, cancer is a disease of cells. The only way to diagnose cancer conclusively is to test a sample of the abnormal cells. The usual way of doing this is to obtain a **biopsy**. All this means is examining a small sample of tissue by one method or another. Before a biopsy is performed, the doctor will ask a series of questions to try and find out the cause of the symptoms. There is no specific symptom of cancer; it depends on where the tumour is, how big it is, which structures it is invading and whether it has spread to other parts of the body. A patient with lung cancer, for example, may have a cough, sometimes with blood or phlegm, or a persistent chest infection that does not respond to antibiotics. Non-specific symptoms such as fatigue, weight loss, loss of appetite and depression can also occur. The usual symptom of breast cancer is a lump in the breast, although it may well spread before it can be detected in this way. If it does so, the symptoms it produces will depend on the site to which it spreads. If it spreads to the lungs, then it may mimic a lung tumour; if it goes to the liver, a liver tumour and so on. Cancer of the cervix can cause abnormal bleeding between periods or persistent bleeding in women who have already reached the menopause; patients suffering from colon cancer may have abdominal pain, diarrhoea or blood in the stools. Every symptom that cancer produces can be mimicked by completely benign and harmless conditions. Just as a chest infection can mimic lung cancer, most lumps in the breast are not due to cancer. If the symptoms are not controlled by straightforward medication of the sort usually available in every household, then you should consult your GP who will decide what further tests are necessary.

The first thing a doctor will do is examine you, noting your pulse, temperature and sometimes blood pressure. He will examine your chest and abdomen, listening for abnormal function of the lungs and feeling for abnormal masses in the liver, spleen and other abdominal organs. Blood tests to see if you are anaemic or have a low white blood cell count, and tests for kidney and liver function may be carried out. A chest X-ray and more specific tests may be requested depending on the likely site of the primary tumour. There is a whole range of investigations that can be performed. At this stage, the GP may already have a good idea of what is wrong, and will refer you to a surgeon at hospital, so that a biopsy can be performed. If cancer is diagnosed, you will usually see a specialist for further treatment.

Sometimes the diagnosis can be made without a biopsy. A diagnosis of lung cancer can be made by seeing abnormal cells in sputum coughed into a container and examined microscopically. Similarly, if fluid has gathered in the cavity surrounding the intestines, then simply putting a needle in – a relatively painless process – and removing a few drops of fluid can provide a diagnosis. In most cases, however, the surgeon will obtain a biopsy under anaesthetic.

Diagnosing cancer

- Blood tests can check for anaemia, bone marrow function, how the liver and kidneys are working.
- Some cancers secrete substances which can be detected in the blood.
- Plain X-rays provide information about various parts of the body.
- Contrast X-rays, performed by giving an injection or drink of a substance that will show up on the X-ray, can be more useful.
- CT (computerised tomography) scans can provide detailed information about the structure of various organs.
- Bone and liver scans can show areas of defective function perhaps caused by a tumour.
- A biopsy – the sampling of a piece of tissue thought to contain the cancer – is the definitive way to make the diagnosis.

BIOPSY

Usually the only sure way to make a diagnosis of cancer is to take a biopsy of the affected part of the body. A biopsy is just a sample of living tissue. If the tumour is very small then it may be completely removed and the whole sample sent to the laboratory for examination. If it is larger then a tiny fragment may be taken.

It is obviously easy to get a sample of tissue from the surface, so samples of skin tumours can be taken under local anaesthetic. This is done in the clinic and takes a few minutes. Antiseptic solution is swabbed over the area to be sampled and, using a very fine needle, local anaesthetic is injected. There is a tiny prick to start with and then the area becomes numb within about twenty seconds. The doctor makes a little nick in the skin with a scalpel and cuts out a small sample. A single stitch is often all that is needed to allow healing. After a few days the wound heals completely, leaving a small scar. In time this disappears.

Tumours that lie deep under the skin are more difficult to get at. A swollen lymph gland in the neck, for example, may wriggle around making biopsy under local anaesthetic uncomfortable. So here the patient is taken to an operating theatre and put to sleep with a general anaesthetic and the procedure carried out painlessly. By doing this the muscles of the body relax, allowing the doctor to get a much better impression of where the tumour really is just by feeling around. Indeed examination under anaesthesia, or E.U.A. for short, is sometimes an essential part of defining how far a tumour has spread.

If the tumour is deep inside the body then there are a variety of ways of obtaining tissue samples. **Endoscopy** (looking inside the body) is the general term for doing this. This involves passing a fine, flexible tube, made of optical fibres, through the body's natural openings to reach the site to be examined and allow a sample of tissue to be removed. Common sites where endoscopy is performed include the oesophagus, stomach, rectum, colon, lungs and peritoneal cavity of the abdomen. Nowadays this can be done under local anaesthetic and is surprisingly painless.

Take endoscopy of the stomach, for example. There is no need to stay the night in hospital for this unless you live a long way away or other tests are going to be done at the same time. You will be asked not to eat anything for several hours beforehand so that your stomach is empty to give the doctor a better view. A sedative injection is given and a tube placed in your mouth and gradually swallowed. When it reaches your stomach the doctor can look down the eyepiece outside and see the inside stomach wall beautifully displayed in full colour. There is a camera attachment so that a full record can be made. You will not be able to see the picture yourself as you are being endoscoped, but if you are interested ask to see the photographs later. There is also a remotely controlled pair of fine tweezers so a biopsy of any suspicious area can be taken. As there are no nerve fibres inside the stomach there is no pain at all when the tweezers are used. This applies to all areas which are endoscoped. The tube is then removed and after a short rest you can go home. The actual procedure only takes a few minutes.

More recently, needle biopsies have been used in certain parts of the body. This sounds like some form of mediaeval torture! In fact, like endoscopy, the whole business is almost painless. Local anaesthetic is used to numb the sensitive nerve fibres lying under the skin. A fine needle 2–10 centimetres long is then passed through the skin into the area thought to contain a tumour. The needle is connected to a syringe which sucks up a few cells from this area. The needle is then withdrawn and the cells are pushed out onto a glass slide for examination under a microscope later. The whole procedure is over in a matter of minutes. Sometimes X-rays are used to make sure the needle is in exactly the right place – for example, when sampling an unusual shadow on a chest X-ray to see if it is lung cancer.

A tissue sample, whether taken by open biopsy, endoscopy or using a fine needle, is then sent to the pathology laboratory for examination. The tissue is then embedded in wax. Sections are then cut using a sharp knife. The sections are layered onto a microscope slide, stained with dyes that will outline the shapes of cells and their nuclei, and reviewed by the pathologist. His job is to assess exactly what is going on in the tissue. His skills are absolutely vital in sorting out whether a particular abnormality is benign or malignant. He does this by recognising patterns in the tissue. With experience, the pathologist can quickly tell the nature of the lesion. This is essential in deciding on the best treatment.

THE ONCOLOGIST

The surgeon who performs the biopsy, and the physician who carries out the various investigations that lead to the diagnosis of cancer, are not usually specialists in the treatment of the disease. Sometimes the surgeon will perform an operation to remove the tumour and that is the only step required. But many patients need other treatment, such as more specialised surgery, radiotherapy or treatment with anti-cancer drugs (chemotherapy). These are all specialised disciplines within medicine. Oncology is the study of tumours. It is derived from the Greek word, *oncos*, meaning a lump. An **oncologist**, therefore, is a doctor who specialises in the treatment of patients with cancer.

To make things more confusing, there are different types of oncologists. A clinical oncologist is the broad term for any doctor who specialises in the care of cancer patients. A surgical oncologist is a surgeon. A radiotherapist – sometimes known as a radiation oncologist – is involved in the use of radiotherapy. A medical oncologist specialises in the treatment of cancer with drugs.

Although cancer is common, many smaller hospitals do not have a full-time oncologist. Instead, a cancer specialist will visit from a larger centre on a weekly or fortnightly basis to run a clinic and see new patients. He may also do a ward round.

A word about the hospital hierarchy. The consultant is the specialist responsible for your care. Underneath him there will be a team of doctors including senior registrars, registrars, senior house officers and house officers in descending order of experience. In a cancer centre all the doctors in the team will specialise in the treatment of cancer. In smaller hospitals, the team may have a much more general function dealing with many common illnesses. If you are unclear as to what is going on you should seek advice from the consultant about the overall strategy of your care.

By the time you see a cancer specialist, the diagnosis will have been made. Drawing up a plan for your treatment is the next step. For many curable cancers, it is vital that this plan is tailored to the individual. The best chance of cure lies in getting the correct treatment as early as possible.

The first thing the cancer specialist will do is ask questions and examine you. He will then review the investigations that have been performed and perhaps request more. The reason for this is that he is seeing you in a different light. He wants to get as much information as possible about the tumour and you, so that tumour growth can be followed easily. This may mean more blood tests to look for substances produced by the tumour and secreted into the blood or special X-rays such as computerised scans to determine how big a tumour is at a particular site. If there is any doubt as to the diagnosis, you may even need a further biopsy, although this is extremely rare. The specialist uses all this information to assess how far the disease has spread. This process is called **staging**.

STAGING

Many staging systems have evolved over the last few decades. These are a useful way of comparing the results of different treatments in different centres.

One of the most commonly used staging systems is the TNM system which was developed by a committee of the UICC (International Union Against Cancer). In this system, the letter T stands for tumour; T1 implies a small tumour and T4 a very large tumour. Other numbers and letters are added to the T numbers to denote different sites of the body. For example, N stands for nodes – the lymph nodes draining the organ in which the tumour is found. Enlarged nodes containing growing tumours are classified as N2. M stands for metastases (spread of the disease) which are either present (M1) or absent (M0).

By knowing the stage a cancer has reached, the doctor has a good idea of what the patient's chances of recovery are. An early stage (Stage 1) has a better chance of recovering than a late stage (Stage 3 or 4) of the same disease.

In most cancers the treatment will depend on the degree of spread. In Hodgkin's disease, for example, the disease can be treated with local radiotherapy at an early stage; but if it has spread to other areas, chemotherapy is the usual treatment.

The specialist will also look at the information obtained from the biopsy. This sort of information gives the doctor a very good idea of how a tumour is likely to behave. This procedure is called **grading**.

The grade refers to the degree of malignancy (that is, how quickly a tumour is spreading). High-grade tumours are very abnormal and the cell turnover rate is high. As a result they tend to grow rapidly and invade widely. Under the microscope, they can easily be distinguished from the surrounding normal tissue. At the other end of the spectrum, low-grade tumours are relatively similar to the surrounding tissue and have very few cells which are dividing. Such tumours grow more slowly and are less likely to spread early. Since the effectiveness of chemotherapy and radiotherapy depends on interfering with the cell cycle in some way, low-grade tumours, where only a small proportion of the cells are dividing, may be resistant. Conversely, high-grade tumours, in which a high proportion of the cells are dividing, are likely to be most sensitive. Such tumours respond by shrinking rapidly, whilst low-grade tumours shrink more slowly. On the other hand, the latter regrow more slowly whereas high-grade tumours can grow back much more rapidly. Hence the paradox that high-grade, aggressive tumours are more sensitive to treatment. This is only a general guide, however, and there are often exceptions.

A combination of stage and grade provides the specialist with a fair idea of what is likely to happen, and can be used to decide on the best treatment for that particular patient.

X-RAY INVESTIGATIONS

X-rays are often used as quick diagnostic tests, either before or after the biopsy. The most common X-ray is that of the chest. This provides information about the size of the heart, the presence of tumours in the lungs or in the lymph nodes at the centre of the chest, and also whether any of the bone structure of the ribs and spine has been infiltrated by tumour. X-rays yield information because they penetrate tissues differently, producing images of bone, lungs, fat and so on. But while they are very good for detecting broken bones, they are not so good for looking at subtle changes in the soft tissues of the body. Although a 2 cm lung tumour is visible on a chest X-ray, a 2 cm colon tumour cannot be seen on an abdominal X-ray. There is little difference between the water content of a tumour in the abdomen and the surrounding tissue.

Newer X-ray technology has been developed to get over this problem. Over the last ten years, computerised tomographic (CT) scans have become widespread. CT scanners are often known as cancer scanners, although they have many more uses than just detecting cancer. When having a scan, the patient lies on a table for about forty-five minutes while a huge revolving disc moves up and down, taking X-rays. A computer calculates the tissue density at many defined sites in the body. In this way, the scanner produces a series of slices outlining internal structures based on their different water content. The whole procedure is completely painless. CT scans are extremely useful in measuring the size of the tumour and assessing how far a tumour has spread, particularly in the abdomen.

X-ray examinations can also be performed using contrast fluid. This allows the structure of various internal organs to be seen more clearly. The most common contrast study is the barium meal. Here you will be given a chalky white fluid containing barium sulphate to drink after fasting for four hours. Your stomach should be empty after this time so the barium flows freely around the inner lining. The barium can be seen on an X-ray screen and pictures taken of any suspicious areas. The fluid is not exactly champagne to drink but, despite all rumours, it doesn't taste too bad. The doctor performing the investigation may put you in unusual positions so the barium can swirl around in the stomach to give the best pictures and show up any irregularity. Sometimes the X-rays are good enough to determine the diagnosis but often a biopsy is needed for confirmation.

Ultrasound is a completely painless procedure in which sound waves are sent into the body and their echoes recorded and used to build an image of the body cavities. For this procedure some jelly is rubbed on the skin and a metal probe placed over the relevant area. Tumours in the abdomen and pelvis can often be identified and their growth pattern followed using this method. It is also used in pregnancy to monitor the growth of the foetus – so it is very safe. More recently magnetic resonance imaging (MRI), another technique which does not use X-rays, has been introduced. In some areas, for example the brain and the pelvis, images produced by MRI are of better quality than CT.

Not all patients have these complex and expensive investigations. The reason for this is not meanness on the part of the consultant responsible. Diagnostic tests are only done if they are going to help in the choice of treatment by giving valuable information on the size of the tumour and how far it has spread. It is interesting to compare the number of tests performed here in a British NHS hospital with those at a private hospital in the United States. The whole basis of hospital care in the US depends on a high turnover of investigations. Without this, the hospital would go bust.

For this reason, most patients in the US are over-investigated. So don't feel that you're not getting proper treatment if you're not given lots of tests.

PRIVATE MEDICINE AND CANCER

A growing number of patients are being treated privately, either paying their fees directly or through one of the medical insurance companies. More and more employers use insurance schemes as a perk for senior staff. GP care is usually through the NHS but tests to diagnose cancer may be performed privately. A decision then has to be made about treatment.

The first thing to note is that private health care is very expensive. There is no rip-off – it's just that the true cost of all health care is high. The fact that the NHS is free makes many of us undervalue its services. The amount of money we spend as a nation per year on health care is low and the NHS is a surprisingly efficient structure. One of the reasons for this is the quality of our GP service. This streamlines patients into the relevant services. In many countries where GPs do not exist, patients go running round various specialists having what is often called a 'wallet biopsy'. Sadly, this still goes on in certain areas of the private sector in the UK. If you are contemplating private care and have not got insurance, note the costs involved, especially those involving hospital stay. Hospitals are expensive places to run. The

Costs of private care

	£
Hospital bed per night	200–400
Intensive care (per night)	800
Initial consultation	50–100
Simple X-rays and blood tests	15 each
CT scan	150–250
Bone scan	75
Biopsy evaluation by pathologist	45
Surgery for colon cancer	2000
Radiotherapy for breast cancer	2000
Chemotherapy for testis cancer	5000

cost of a bed in a rather depressing Victorian workhouse, which passes as a cancer ward in some NHS hospitals, with nursing, drugs, medical staff and administration runs to about £250 per day. As you can see from the table, many so-called 'hospital plans', which pay so much a day when you go to hospital, come nowhere near providing the amount required for private treatment. These costs can only be approximate as there is considerable variation depending on where the procedures are carried out. Private hospital care in London is by far the most expensive.

The most important thing about cancer treatment is that the correct decision is made at each step about the best possible plan for therapy. The environment in which this is done is irrelevant. Many leading cancer centres operate under very primitive conditions and many charlatans practise in the elegant portals of Harley Street. How can the consumer know what is best in the private sector?

The first thing to ensure is that your specialist really is a consultant. Many doctors with minimum qualifications are practising as pseudo-specialists in London. They may have no hospital appointment and are really little more than crooks. They tend to work with patients from overseas who are grateful to be seen by anybody even for exorbitant fees. Make sure your specialist has an NHS appointment as a consultant. Your public library will have a Medical Directory in which you can look up his qualifications. If you are in any doubt, talk to your own GP who should be able to guide you through the specialist care currently available. The main attractions of going privately are the quality of the 'hotel' services offered when in hospital and the fact that you will see your consultant on nearly every occasion. Within the NHS you may be seen by several doctors, some of whom will be learning their speciality. This actually allows for greater safety, surprising as this might seem. Young doctors are much more questioning and will discuss any problems eagerly with their consultants. Thus, there will be a greater pool of knowledge around from several sources. At the end of the day, the X-rays in radiotherapy and the drugs given for chemotherapy are going to be the same.

Cancer care in the UK compares very favourably with that of most developed nations. One weak spot has been the failure to develop centres of excellence of an adequate size. This means that there are still many small units staffed by one or two specialists who may well be near to retirement and not up-to-date on the latest methods of treatment. The equipment may be antiquated. If you are worried, ask your GP to refer you to a larger centre, such as that associated with a teaching hospital. Even though the travelling distance may be greater it may well be worth it in the long term.

You are also entitled to a second opinion in the NHS. This means your doctor can refer you to any other specialist of his choice to assess you, review your investigations and decide if the planned treatment is appropriate. Specific recommendations are often made during second opinions. You need not worry that your doctor will be offended if you want a second opinion. If he is then it is probably just as well you are asking. It may be a sign of his insecurity and perhaps even lack of knowledge.

Assessing Your Chances of Being Cured

When treatment is being given, there are standard methods of assessing what is happening. A 'complete response' means that the tumour has disappeared completely; a 'partial response' that it has shrunk by 50 per cent of its area on an X-ray or by some other measure; and 'no response' means nothing has happened.

Unfortunately, it is not just whether a tumour responds to treatment that determines whether it can be cured. If it comes back at its original site or elsewhere, the patient will develop further problems. The best way to assess the cure rate for cancer is to look at survival curves (Figure 3.2). If we treat 100 patients with lung cancer and look at their survival, it is very clear that they do much less well than those of the same age that did not have the cancer. To define cure we have to show that the survival rate of a cured group of patients is the same as those *of similar age and sex* that did not have cancer in the first place. Usually, this is measured after five years. Thus, the five-year percentage survival is a good indicator of the number of patients likely to be cured. Unfortunately, for some cancers this is not the case. In

Doctors' qualifications

MB BS
MB BChir
MB BCh
Bachelor of Medicine and Bachelor of Surgery. These are the basic medical qualifications given by British universities.

LMSSA
LRCP
MRCS
Diplomas of no greater value than the above basic qualifications. The examinations for them are often a bit easier, so these may well be held by those having problems in passing their university finals. There are many other diplomas which require only a few months' postgraduate study and are really of little value. These are readily displayed by some private sector doctors who hope you will judge them by counting the number of letters after their name!

MRCP
Membership of the Royal College of Physicians – held by those trained in internal medicine. It is usually converted to a fellowship (FRCP) without further examination some ten years later.

FRCS
Fellowship of the Royal College of Surgeons – a basic surgical qualification given after examination following three to four years' postgraduate study.

FRCR
Fellowship of the Royal College of Radiologists. This requires three years' training in either diagnostic X-rays or radiotherapy. Some older doctors have the FFR – the equivalent qualification given before the College became ' independent. Doctors putting both FRCR and FFR after their name are also in the letter-counting game.

DMRT
Diploma of Medical Radiotherapy, requiring two years' study – really a poor man's FRCR.

MD
Doctor of Medicine. In Britain this is a further degree which requires research and the submission of a thesis. In many other countries such as the US it denotes the basic medical qualification.

PhD
Doctor of Philosophy, given for research and a thesis, usually on a more laboratory-based topic.

ACCREDITATION
Over the last few years, accreditation has been given to those doctors who have spent the necessary time in training posts in either radiotherapy or medical oncology.

breast cancer, for example, patients go on developing recurrent tumours for many years afterwards, although the rate at which this happens slows down as the years pass.

The emphasis on comparing people of similar age is important. We are all dying slowly all the time. The chances of dying increase with age. So a group of school children have a very flat survival curve; and a group of old age pensioners, a much steeper one, even if they do not have cancer. Life assurance companies have collected this type of information and reflect it in the premiums they charge for people of different ages. We also know that some types of cancer are more resistant to treatment in older patients. Using five-year survival to compare treatment in an area where a lot of old age pensioners live, such as Eastbourne, to a new town development, such as Milton Keynes, may be unfair to Eastbourne doctors unless age is corrected for in the calculations.

GETTING INFORMATION

Just as we are all different in all sorts of ways, we all need different amounts of information about our disease. Some patients are quite content to leave it to the doctors to get on with their treatment plan and not even ask if they have cancer. Indeed, some go as far as denying they have cancer even though they have been told the diagnosis on several occasions. Other patients want to know everything down to the last detail and wish to be involved in treatment decisions. Doctors have now come to respect patient preferences, and most cancer specialists have an open mind, answering questions honestly and as best they can. But to get the information you want you must know what to ask. Many people are unfamiliar with the workings of a motor car, but are quite happy to nod wisely whilst a mechanic explains in technical terms and come away with only a vague idea of what is wrong. As long as it can be fixed at a reasonable price, does it matter anyway? But if you or a close relative or friend has cancer, there is more at stake than a car; after all, a car can always be replaced.

This book will give you a good grasp of the processes involved in cancer care. If you are diagnosed as having cancer, you will want to know what type of tumour it is, what the primary site is, where it has spread, its stage and perhaps other information that can give you clues as to the likely chances of being cured. Do not be afraid to ask; many doctors will not volunteer much information unless probed by the patient. There are still many physicians who adopt a rather paternalistic attitude, patting the patient on the back and telling them not to worry. This may also cover up a doctor's ignorance and his indecision as to what to do. Probe for the answers. We know from experience in the clinic that those patients who ask will receive information, and those who do not may not get it. Many young doctors beginning in oncology are very good at explaining things to patients. But if you are not getting the answers to your questions ask to see the consultant; he is responsible for your care.

We have made a list of questions which you might like to use. We would stress, however, that it is much better to get them answered during a free-flowing discussion, rather than you giving the consultant a structured interview. Some patients find it helpful to bring recorders to tape the doctor's replies so that they can be listened to again at home. When the diagnosis of cancer is first mentioned, people are often too shocked to ask questions. But cancer treatment is not usually started immediately, so there is plenty of time to think things out and to come back with questions.

Checklist of Questions

- What type of tumour is it?
- How big is the primary tumour?
- Has it spread to the lymph nodes?
- Has it spread anywhere else in the body?
- What stage is the tumour?
- Are there any indications from the pathologist, and are they good or bad?
- What treatment do you propose to carry out?
- Where will this treatment be done and who will be responsible for it?
- Will I have to go into hospital and if so, for how long?
- What are the side-effects of any drugs that I might need?

- How often will the drugs be given and for how long?
- What are the chances of my tumour being cured?
- If it cannot be cured, could you give me a rough idea of my life expectancy?

In this book we do not go into great detail about specific tumours. But in chapter 10 we list a variety of sources where useful information can be obtained on individual cancers. In addition, cancer information services such as BACUP and Cancerlink will provide excellent booklets on specific cancer types. These can be used to help you frame the questions you want answered. As we keep stressing, the quality of the information received is up to you. There are still vestiges of paternalism within the NHS left over from the charity hospital system. These Victorian attitudes have to be cast aside in the consumer age of the late twentieth century and the impetus must come from you.

SECOND OPINION

Doctors often disagree and have done so since the first teachings of Hippocrates. The reason for the disagreement is that medicine is in many ways still an art rather than an exact science: there are several ways in which the same result can be achieved. Cancer medicine is no exception. Many large centres have case conferences where individual patient problems are discussed and a body of opinion can be formed. There is regular disagreement on even the most simple decisions such as whether to recommend post-operative radiotherapy or on how many doses of chemotherapy should be given following an operation.

If you are happy with the information you have received, well and good; but if you are not, you are quite entitled to get a second opinion from another specialist. There is an unwritten rule of medical practice in the UK that patients are not seen by specialists without a request from their GP. The reason for this is sensible. If you turned up to see another specialist, having had a series of investigations and perhaps a biopsy performed elsewhere, the second specialist would have to start again unless they had the results available. The information that many patients have about their condition may not reflect the actual situation because of misunderstandings creeping in at various stages. To get a valuable second opinion, all the information must be laid in front of the specialist. In the US, where second opinions are very costly, the doctor will insist on seeing all the X-rays performed and obtain biopsy material for review by his own pathologist. This is rather extreme, but in difficult cases may be the only way to get a worthwhile consultation. At the very least, a letter from the GP stating the problem, perhaps with a copy of the summary of the first specialist, is essential. No doctor of any standing will be offended if you ask for a second opinion. We all realise the complexity of modern medicine and that no single person can be infallible. Major surgery for cancer can result in a complete change of lifestyle. So feel free to ask for a second opinion.

GETTING THE FACTS FROM YOUR DOCTOR

- Make a list of questions you want answered.
- Do not be afraid to ask anything – the doctor will usually respond truthfully.
- Make sure you know what alternatives are available.
- Take a relative or close friend with you – you can then discuss the answers afterwards.
- Taking a cassette recorder may be helpful but is rather intimidating for the doctor – the answers you get may be much more guarded.
- Discuss any queries with your GP.
- If you are not happy about any aspect of your treatment, tell the doctors.
- Ask to see the consultant responsible for your care if you are unhappy.
- Nurses and radiographers are a very useful source of information.

SURGERY

Surgery is the oldest form of treatment for cancer. The Greeks and Romans were skilled at tumour removal and sometimes cured patients with what would now be regarded as very primitive operations. There were no anaesthetics or antiseptics. Antibiotics to combat post-operative infection were undreamed of, and so the chances of an operation being successful were pretty minimal. Nowadays the position has changed. Surgery has evolved into a scientific discipline in which a detailed knowledge of the structure and function of the body, together with advanced technology of the twentieth century, have resulted in many operations being possible which could not be done before.

The aim of cancer surgery is to remove the whole tumour leaving behind as much of the normal tissue as possible. The cancer surgeon is performing a balancing act. The tumour must be removed in its entirety for the operation to be a success; and yet, if too much normal tissue is taken away with the tumour, the patient may have serious problems. Advances in cancer surgery have come from knowing, with confidence, exactly how much tissue needs to be removed. The history of breast cancer treatment is a very good example of this.

BREAST CANCER

The most usual symptom of breast cancer is a lump in the breast. The majority are small, usually under 5 cm (2 in.) in diameter. Despite their size they may spread through the lymphatic channels into the lymph nodes under the armpits or across the chest into the other armpit, or track up into the lymph nodes in the neck. In addition, small clusters of cells may break off and get carried in the bloodstream to the bones, liver and brain: areas where breast cancer cells like to grow. Different tumours behave in very different ways, and despite some recent interesting information we have no certain way of predicting how a tumour will behave in an individual patient.

Until the late nineteenth century, breast cancer surgery was a very crude affair and used only for the worst types of tumour, well beyond cure. In 1890 William Halstead, an American surgeon working in Baltimore, pioneered an operation that still bears his name – the Halstead radical mastectomy. **Mastectomy** means removal of the breast. Halstead believed that by removing the whole breast, together with the lymph nodes under the armpit and a significant amount of underlying muscle, he would be able to encompass the whole tumour.

For many years, the Halstead method of mastectomy dominated the treatment of breast cancer throughout the world. It seemed logical that removing the draining lymph nodes at the same time as the tumour would increase survival. After all, pathologists at the time could actually see clusters of breast cancer cells in the removed lymph nodes. Surely this must be the best treatment? But removal of the main muscle of the chest left women with considerable deformity: the whole chest became lopsided. It was difficult to correct this completely by any form of prosthesis (a prosthesis is the name for an artificial breast in this instance). The lymphatics were often damaged so that the arm on the same side would swell up even though the patient was cured of her disease.

Dissatisfied with the results, several surgeons during the 1940s decided to try modifications of Halstead's hallowed operation. They no longer removed most of the main muscle covering the rib cage. Years later, the results of this new operation were compared to the Halstead procedure and found to be the same. The new operation was widely adopted.

At the same time Geoffrey Keynes, a radiotherapist working at St Thomas's Hospital, was pioneering work with radioactive implants. His results suggested that mastectomy might not be necessary in all patients. During the 1950s, radiotherapy improved still further with the advent of new higher-energy machines to deliver radiation – linear accelerators and cobalt units. For the first time radiation could be given in a predictable and tailored manner, following the contours of the body without causing excessive damage in areas receiving the highest doses. Various clinical trials were set up to establish if radiotherapy to the chest wall and lymph nodes draining the breast would be of any value after radical mastectomy.

In addition, surgeons began to experiment with more conservative types of treatment. A simple mastectomy was the next operation. This involved removing the breast but not the lymph nodes or muscle. For women with small lumps and no evidence of disease under the armpit, it produced exactly the same results as the radical mastectomy. In the early 1970s, this was the commonest operation. There was considerable controversy about whether radiotherapy should be given after simple mastectomy. We now know that unless the tumour is large or the lymph nodes are diseased, radiotherapy may not be necessary.

Finally, some surgeons did what in the past would have been unthinkable: they removed only the tumour, leaving the normal breast around it intact. Following this, patients were given radiotherapy with a small booster dose to the tumour bed. When results were compared to those of patients who had received other types of treatment, the percentage of survivors was exactly the same.

Women who have conservative treatment, often referred to as lumpectomy (the removal of the lump), followed by radiotherapy, are usually very satisfied with the results. Psychologically, many women prefer to be left with apparently normal breasts. However, individuals vary widely and the possible options should always be fully discussed with the doctor in charge of the case. Given the choice, Nancy Reagan had a mastectomy. In the case of lumpectomy, the only change that can be seen is the absence of hair under the armpit on the irradiated side. If the lump is small and the surgeon skilled at producing a good cosmetic result, it is often difficult for the doctor in the follow-up clinic to tell which breast has been involved.

Many clinical studies have now proved the wisdom of a conservative surgical approach. How can these results be explained? Surely more aggressive surgery, removing lymph nodes and underlying muscle, stands to produce greater gains in terms of cure? The reason why it does not is that lymph nodes do not act as a barrier to breast cancer spread. However radical the surgery, it cannot deal with small clumps of cells in other organs of the body. If the disease has already spread at the time of surgery, then removing the lymph nodes and underlying tissue will be no use. These patients will definitely have a recurrence of the disease, whatever surgery or radiotherapy is given. Therefore, moving to conservative treatments makes perfect sense.

But not all patients are suited for this type of approach. Elderly patients, for example, often have small breasts and may have a large tumour. They are still better treated with mastectomy. There are many other reasons why a more extensive operation may be indicated. If the tumour is central and the remaining breast is likely to be small with no nipple, it may be preferable to have the breast removed and be able to wear a prosthesis comfortably.

Clearly it is your right as a patient to know exactly what is going on and why. Surgeons are often not the best communicators. As elsewhere in this book, we urge you to ask what is happening. After all, it is your body. For every operation a consent form must be signed. It will say that the procedure to be carried out has been fully explained to you. Do not sign it unless you are happy with the information you have received.

COLORECTAL CANCER

Cancer of the colon, like breast cancer, is a common disease. It is called colorectal because the majority of colon tumours are at the lower end of the colon, which blends into the rectum – the opening of the bowel to the outside. Colorectal tumours usually result in blood in the stool, the production of excess mucus, occasional abdominal pain and sometimes diarrhoea. Any persistent change of bowel habit should be reported to your doctor who will perform the necessary investigations.

Those tumours that are high in the colon can be removed through an operation in which the abdominal wall is opened from the front, the tumour cut out and the pieces of intestine joined together. This procedure is called an anterior resection (literally, cutting the tumour out from the front). A problem faces the surgeon when the tumour is at the lower end of the colon or within the rectum. If he is to cut enough tissue to destroy the disease, he may destroy the mechanism which controls bowel movement. The standard procedure for these operations until ten years ago was to perform a **colostomy** – to remove the affected bowel (without being able to conserve the anal sphincter) and provide the patient with a bag. It is usually easy to adapt to this, but it is better avoided if possible.

The advent of a new piece of surgical equipment has changed this radically. The surgeon can cut away tumour at the lower end of the colon and then, by using a staple gun, join the two ends deep inside the pelvis. This means that many more patients are spared the need for a colostomy – a good example of how technology has improved, reducing the need for extensive surgery.

BONE TUMOURS

Bone tumours are relatively rare, but do occur in children and young adults. They usually occur on the leg. In the past, the standard procedure was an amputation above the level of the tumour, usually followed by chemotherapy to destroy any small deposits of tumour cells. Amputating limbs in children is very sad. Children adapt remarkably well, but of course are left with a lifelong legacy of their cancer. For some years now, orthopaedic surgeons have been experimenting with more conservative approaches: removing the bone containing the tumour and putting in artificial bone and usually a metal rod. Alternatively, bone grafts may be used from other parts of the body where bones are not essential, such as the wing of the pelvis. This is the bone that can be felt by pressing down on the hips. These bone wings are not essential to our anatomy. Pieces can be chipped off and inserted in place of a long bone. If all goes well, they will heal and provide a perfectly functional bone in the leg or arm. The use of radiotherapy and chemotherapy at the same time means that the end result, in terms of the number of patients cured, is exactly the same as with amputation. Most childhood bone tumours are now treated in this way.

THE OPERATION

Having a cancer operation is really like any other. You usually come into the hospital a day or so before the operation so that any last-minute investigations can be performed. Your general condition will be assessed to make sure there is no chest infection as this can cause complications after the anaesthetic. The first doctor you see is the house surgeon. He or she is the most junior member of the team and will ask questions, give you a thorough examination and organise the various tests. You may then be seen by the anaesthetist to make sure you are not on any medication that might interact with the anaesthetic.

On the day of the operation you will be given pre-medication (an injection or tablets) to make you feel comfortable and less nervous before going to the operating theatre. In a side room of the theatre, the anaesthetic is given. This is a completely painless and not unpleasant process – a simple injection into your arm will send you to sleep within ten seconds. Then the operation begins. After the operation, you will spend some time in a recovery area where your heart and breathing are monitored closely to make sure you have recovered fully from the anaesthetic. Then you will be taken back to the ward.

The length of time spent in hospital depends on the type of operation carried out and whether there are any medical problems such as heart disease, chest infection, diabetes and so on. The removal of a breast lump may only require overnight admission. A major abdominal operation for the removal of a lung for lung cancer may mean staying in hospital for two to three weeks. Over the last decade, it has become recognised more and more that bed is a dangerous place to be after surgery. The surgical team and nurses will encourage you to move around as much as possible. This is to get the blood moving in the veins to prevent any clotting. This post-operative bullying by staff is all for your own good and should not be regarded as unpleasantness! During this period, you may meet radiotherapy and chemotherapy specialists to sort out the next stage in your treatment. Before leaving hospital it is important to make sure arrangements have been made for follow-up. Not everybody requires treatment other than surgery. But most will come back to the clinic regularly for check-ups and perhaps to have certain investigations.

CONVALESCENCE

Not so long ago, most large hospitals had convalescent homes associated with them, usually by the seaside. The patient would be sent there to convalesce for two to three weeks. This really meant protracted rest, sitting around, lounging and getting very bored. We now know that it is much better for patients, both physically and psychologically, to get back to their own environment, and indeeed to their normal activity as soon as possible. Cancer surgery is no exception. For this reason most of the convalescent homes have disappeared. Many patients are back to work within a few days of an operation. Obviously there are exceptions, especially if problems occur after the operation. A busy mother with three or four children to look after may find it rather difficult to cope after a major operation, and allowances must be made. The best advice about convalescence is to do as much as possible, but stop when tiredness takes over.

PRIVATE SURGERY

The biggest advantage in private surgery is that you will deal with one person, the consultant surgeon. There will be very few others involved in decisions about your care during the time of operation. By going privately you will have more flexibility about when to have the operation, and your time with the consultant will probably be in more relaxed surroundings. You will be able to discuss the whole problem and, obviously, have the operation carried out in a private hospital or private wing of an NHS hospital. Private hospitals are usually more attractive, with such trimmings as carpets on the floor, television by every bed, telephones, single rooms and better quality of food.

Despite all this, there is not one shred of evidence that private medicine actually produces better results than the NHS. Although the 'hotel facilities' (room service, food and surroundings) vary enormously, the quality of medical and nursing care is remarkably high throughout Britain. It is for this reason that the end results do not differ. If you decide to go privately, do not look on it as buying you a ticket for a cure. Regard it like first class on a train. First- and second-class passengers get to the same place at the same time. It is just the quality of the surroundings that is different.

If everything is straightforward, private medicine has no disadvantages, but if something goes wrong following the operation, perhaps in the middle of the night, you may be much better off in an NHS hospital. The resident doctors there are more likely to have expertise in the problem you have, and be better equipped to deal with any emergency, than in a small private hospital. Indeed, there are some tiny little nursing homes in which fairly major surgery is now performed by surgeons who should know better.

By tradition, surgical operations attract enormous fees compared with the cost of the hospital or nursing home. If the costs seem enormous, they are! But these are often the true costs of the procedure, even when carried out in an NHS hospital. A bed in a London teaching hospital today costs around £250 per day to run. The table on page 80 lists the likely costs of several surgical operations for cancer. There is enormous variation. If you are paying the fees yourself, do not be afraid to ascertain costs beforehand. The surgeon's secretary or receptionist will usually be able to help. If you belong to one of the insurance companies, such as BUPA or Private Patients' Plan, check that the operation will be carried out on the policy and that no supplement will be necessary. Some surgeons may charge more than the maximum permitted by the insurance company, giving a hefty bill for the treatment. This is often the case in London where much private practice comes from abroad with patients willing to pay exorbitant sums for small operations.

Fees for common cancer operations

Figures include hospital costs

	£
Removal of breast lump	1000
Removal of colon tumour	3000
Removal of lung tumour	5000
Skin tumour excision	500
Biopsy of larynx	500

After a private operation, you may well be referred for radiotherapy or chemotherapy. If you wish to have this on the NHS, this is perfectly permissible. As you will see in later chapters, there is little advantage in private radiotherapy, other than the personal contact with the consultant. Even for chemotherapy, there is little difference. Many patients who go privately value the time they get with the consultant explaining to them and their relatives what is happening. This should be the case in the NHS. Those who ask will receive in most cases. Don't be afraid to do so; after all, it is your health and your body.

THE FUTURE

It is unlikely that any surgical advance is going to result in increased cures for cancer patients. Instead, new techniques providing images of tumours and how far they have spread are being developed and this information will be used by surgeons to delineate the boundaries of the tumour and to minimise damage to normal tissue. As we go into the next decade, it is likely that cancer surgery will become a much more precise science. The development of computerised tomography (CT) scanning has already helped enormously. Some of the new imaging technologies outlined in chapter 9 will take this process further.

Another development which has been watched with great interest by oncologists is organ transplantation. After all, it seems logical that if disease is present in the liver, then the complete removal of the liver followed by a transplant, could be curative. Unfortunately, the results of liver, kidney, pancreas and lung transplantation in cancer patients have been poor. If the tumour is so large that the whole organ needs to be removed, then it is likely to have spread already to other parts of the body. For this reason, it is unlikely that transplant surgery will offer increased hope in the future. Instead, targeting radiotherapy and drugs at cancer cells (thereby sparing normal cells) following operations will increase the number of patients cured. The dramatic improvement in the results of a variety of childhood cancers where surgery is used to remove the tumour is one of the pointers to the future for adults. These children have done remarkably well and many are now healthy and completely cured of their disease. Here the integrated approach, using surgery to take away the bulk of the tumour and radiation and drugs to mop up any cell remnants, has clearly been successful. This is the key for the future of surgery.

S   U   R   G   E   R   Y   –   T   H   E   F   A   C   T   S

- Most patients with cancer have some sort of operation – perhaps just a biopsy.
- There is a lot of controversy about the best type of operation for certain cancers – make sure you understand the alternatives.
- The period of convalescence afterwards varies enormously.
- Private surgery is expensive – make sure you know the costs.
- If insured make sure all the fees will be covered.
- Do not sign the consent form unless you are completely satisfied.

RADIOTHERAPY

Radiotherapy, as a form of treatment for cancer, cannot be considered in isolation. The vast majority of patients with cancer will at some point require surgery, which may entail a simple biopsy or a major operation. In addition, chemotherapy may well form part of treatment either before, during, or after radiotherapy. This combined approach is important and, with greater experience and improved methods of treatment, has led to better results and an improved chance of survival.

Radiotherapy is given by means of X-rays, which were discovered by Wilhelm Roentgen in 1895. Within a year they had been used in the treatment of cancer. We have come a long way since then. The use of radiotherapy in the treatment of cancer is becoming increasingly sophisticated.

WHAT IS RADIOTHERAPY?

The first apparatus for therapeutic X-ray production was invented in the early part of this century by an American named Coolidge. The principles have not changed greatly since then. A heated metal filament produces a beam of electrons which are directed towards a metal plate. When the electrons strike the plate, part of the energy they lose is converted into X-rays which are diverted at high speeds. The amount of energy carried by the X-rays depends on the force with which the electron beam hits the plate and can be altered. The greater the energy of the X-rays, the further they can penetrate into tissue.

Laboratory evidence suggests that radiotherapy works by damaging the DNA in the nucleus of each cell. DNA is a structure which consists of two spirals intertwined. The various parts of the DNA molecule are arranged in a particular sequence – a vital code for proteins which have important functions both inside and outside the cell. Radiation breaks the backbone of the molecule and, when the strands join back together, this vital code is altered. It is this break in the DNA that results in a cell's death. It may be possible for the cell to divide once or twice after exposure to radiation, but eventually all the cells which have been exposed will stop dividing and disintegrate.

Radiotherapy aims to damage malignant cells irreparably whilst limiting the damage to normal tissue in the vicinity. Tumour cells, which usually multiply more frequently than the surrounding normal cells, seem to be more sensitive to radiation and also less likely to be able to repair the damage caused. We have learnt how to exploit this and establish a fine balance between tumour control and damage to normal tissue. In deciding how much radiotherapy to give to a particular tumour, doctors have to set the benefits of treatment against the risk of developing complications. The problem with this approach is that for any individual not only can the risk of complications vary but also their acceptability. Loss of voice will be of greater concern to an opera singer than to a butcher.

DIFFERENT TYPES OF X-RAY TREATMENT

The wonders of modern radiation therapy have only been achieved at the expense of trial and error early in this century. X-rays were discovered by their ability to blacken photographic film and 'X' was used by Roentgen to stand for 'unknown'. The early low-energy X-rays produced dramatic responses in skin cancers where results were easy to see. This led to the use of radiotherapy in a wide range of conditions, including tuberculosis, peptic ulcers and other skin diseases. Although these conditions were untreatable by any other method at the time, a proportion of the patients died as a result of an X-ray overdose and many suffered needlessly. We now know that highly penetrating X-rays, if not monitored and kept below a limit, are far from harmless and for this reason radiotherapy is rarely used except to treat malignant disease. Yet, as recently as the 1950s it was possible to have feet X-rayed in a shoe shop to establish whether or not shoes fitted. It seems inconceivable now, but it was even possible for a child to sit on his pregnant mother's lap whilst having his scalp irradiated for ringworm! But the greatest successes from the use of radiation therapy were seen in the treatment of cancer.

From the outset there were two complementary approaches to treating cancer. One was to use an external radiation source (either X-rays produced by a machine or a radioactive source held at a distance from the patient) and the other a form of treatment where the radioactive source was placed inside the patient. The latter involves implanting radioactive materials, which emit radiation spontaneously as they decay, into the tumour in the form of needles or similar devices. Alternatively, a container with the radioactive source inside may be placed within a cavity such as the uterus – this is known as **interstitial** or **intracavitary radiation**. The use of implanted radioactive sources has been particularly effective in the treatment of cancer of the womb and cervix. In early cancers it may be the only necessary form of radiation, although more commonly it is used in addition to external beam radiotherapy to give an extra high dose to the immediate vicinity of the tumour.

The first radioactive source used for the treatment of cancer was radium. More recently, however, radium has been replaced by other sources, such as caesium, cobalt and iridium. These are preferable both in terms of their powers of penetration, and also in that there is no risk of inhaling radioactive gases. The dose received by the public and staff at a distance from the patient is relatively small. Increasingly stringent rules governing radiation mean that those who come into contact with the patient will be exposed to only a minimal risk. Any risk should be taken seriously, but current knowledge suggests that the chance of such a small radiation exposure resulting in illness or death at a later stage is extremely small. (Far smaller than the risk of cancer from living with a smoker.) The only exceptions are in the exposure of pregnant women or children under the age of about twelve. Children and unborn babies are particularly susceptible to the effects of radiation, and their access to wards where radioactive sources are present is restricted.

Improvements in the last two decades mean that many of the unwanted effects of treatment seen with older, less powerful machinery are now a thing of the past. Indeed, with the advent of a computer for planning as well as CT scanning, it is possible to treat a localised deep-seated tumour with only a slight early skin reaction, and no visible long-term effects in the form of broken blood vessels and skin fibrosis. This is because the high-energy beams currently available are able to penetrate the body more effectively.

Who Is in Charge of Your Treatment?

The first person you are likely to come into contact with is the radiotherapy doctor. With current alterations in the distribution of doctors in different grades, this person is increasingly likely to be a consultant. The consultant takes overall responsibility and will play a large part in deciding what treatment you receive.

The next two ranks in the hierarchy are the senior registrar and registrar. Not all hospitals will have both. If everything goes smoothly, it is likely that both during treatment and in follow-up clinics the registrar will be your main contact. The registrar or senior registrar may well plan your treatment, often supervised by the consultant, and will see you regularly during treatment on a weekly or two-weekly basis and whenever there are problems. The registrar is also likely to be the person corresponding with your GP or referring consultant.

The house officer or senior house officer is the junior doctor who is usually responsible for inpatient care. If you are admitted to the ward for any reason, it is the house officer who will take down your details, examine you and arrange the appropriate investigations. During the ward round, the major decision-making time for your team of doctors, the house officer will relay all the information relating to your case to both the registrars and the consultant.

When you are actually receiving radiotherapy, you will be seen on a daily basis by the radiographers. The radiographers are responsible for setting up the machines, making sure that the correct dose is given and consulting the doctors if they are unhappy about any aspect of your general health during treatment. The need for accuracy here is so great that at least three radiographers will be involved. These will be of varying ranks, with one radiographer taking overall responsibility for a machine. Radiographers are highly qualified individuals who have had at least four years' training and many more years' experience before they are promoted within the hierarchy. They are very knowledgeable and provide a valuable point of contact on a day-to-day basis.

You may not meet the physicists during your treatment but they play a very important part in any radiotherapy department, not least in checking the machines and providing the doctors with the information they need on the distribution of the dose. The physicists also help the doctor decide what form of treatment should be used, given the size and location of any particular tumour.

Although there has been adverse publicity recently, radiotherapy is a remarkably safe form of treatment. There are very clear guidelines on the calibration of machinery, and it is a legal requirement for machines to be checked frequently.

PLANNING

Having decided which treatment is best, the next stage will be to plan it in detail. It is at this stage that you will make your first trip to the radiotherapy centre. X-rays and scans will be taken to determine where the X-ray beam should enter your body. Planning is then carried out on a machine known as the simulator – a machine which literally simulates your treatment on the X-ray therapy machine and can produce X-rays like those used for diagnosis. The position of light beams will then be marked on your skin with a pen. When treating complicated areas where marks are unsightly or less likely to stay, a perspex shell will be made, contoured to fit your body. The purpose of this is to prevent you moving during treatment so that the X-ray beam touches only those tissues it is supposed to touch. Holes are cut out of the shell so that your eyes, nose and mouth are not covered. Marks showing where the X-ray beams should penetrate can then be made on the perspex. Careful notes are kept so that the position of the X-ray beam is the same on each visit you make.

There are standard treatments for certain cancers, but these have to be modified to take into account factors such as your shape, physical mobility, general health, age, sex, the cosmetic result wanted, and even the distance you have to travel for treatment. No two individuals are the same. So don't be alarmed if you compare notes with other patients with the same disease and discover that their treatment is different from yours. There are all sorts of reasons for this, ranging from the stage the disease has reached to personal circumstances such as whether or not it is convenient for you to stay overnight in hospital. If you are at all worried by anything, ask your doctor.

When you initially attend for planning, you will meet at least one doctor, and probably more than one radiographer. Do not be afraid to ask questions about your particular treatment and any fears you may have. On page 88 there is a list of questions you might want to ask when starting radiotherapy.

WHAT IS IT LIKE TO HAVE RADIOTHERAPY?

Once the doctors, radiographers and physicists are satisfied that the treatment prescribed is appropriate and practicable, the treatment will be carried out. The machine used may be a linear accelerator, a machine containing a radioactive source such as cobalt or caesium, or a superficial X-ray machine (used for skin cancers). These are often found in the basement of the building. The machines lie in lead-lined rooms which are built to protect the radiographers and staff outside the room from receiving more than a tiny dose – usually less than one millionth of the dose prescribed for the patient. Different centres will have different machines available, with large

RADIOTHERAPY CHECKLIST

- When will the treatment be planned?
- How long will this take?
- When will the treatment start?
- How many treatments will I have and how long will they last?
- Will it be every day or not?
- Can I drive myself and if so where can I park my car?
- Is hospital transport possible if I feel too ill?
- Can I choose the time I will be treated each day?
- Are there any days when I will not be treated – e.g. public holidays?
- Are there any immediate side effects?
- What should I do about them?
- Is there anything to avoid – e.g. sunbathing, swimming, washing?
- When will I next see the doctor?
- What happens when I finish treatment?

centres having a wider choice. It may be appropriate for the patient to be treated at a smaller centre which is nearer home and does not necessitate hours spent travelling to and from the hospital each day. Once again a cost benefit evaluation has to be performed in which the patient and doctor are involved. If the most important aspect of treatment is the cosmetic result then this may necessitate a lengthy treatment given at a relatively low dose rate in the hope of avoiding skin damage. However, if the final appearance is not of concern, but there are other factors involved (for example a disabled spouse is being left alone for long periods during the day), then a short course of radiotherapy at a higher dose rate may be more appropriate. Radiotherapy is flexible and it is important that the patient makes his or her needs apparent at the outset, so that the doctor can tailor the treatment appropriately.

CURE OR CONTROL?

It is important for people to understand why they are being given radio-therapy. It may be intended as a complete cure – this is known as **radical radiotherapy**. It may be being used to decrease the likelihood of the tumour coming back at the site of origin. A third and very important use of radiotherapy is palliation – to control symptoms. As a general guideline, palliative courses of radiotherapy tend to be shorter.

Radiotherapy may be given as an alternative to surgery. In head and neck cancer, for example, surgery may be more disfiguring than radio-therapy. It may be used after surgery, as in the case of breast cancer; and it may be used before surgery to reduce the size of the tumour so that the operation does not have to be so extensive. In all of these situations, the aim is to reduce the number of cancer cells. Where a cure is hoped for, this would leave no cells capable of forming a further tumour.

The aim of radiotherapy is to treat patients so that the tumour is dam-aged as much as possible while the normal tissue is spared. People who are potentially curable will be treated 'radically' to ensure the best possible cosmetic result and the maximum sparing of normal tissue whilst giving the greatest chance of tumour control. At the other end of the spectrum, a patient who is unlikely to live for a normal period of life and may indeed only be expected to live for weeks or months, will be treated 'palliatively', to control the symptoms. Doctors have to strike a balance between the need for treatment, the time involved and the likely remaining life span.

The majority of tumours are treated with radical radiation over a period of five to six weeks. This is certainly true for tumours in the head and neck, abdomen and pelvis. Four to five weeks' treatment is usually adequate for particularly sensitive tumours such as lymphomas, or particularly radio-resistant tumours, such as melanomas, where large doses of radiotherapy per session of treatment are thought more effective.

One important form of palliative radiotherapy is the 'hemibody' (i.e. half of the body). This can be used to treat patients with widespread secondary spread in the skin or bone where pain is likely to be the main symptom. The patient is admitted to hospital and the area to be treated determined. This may be the lower half of the body from the navel to knees, or the upper half of the body from the navel up to the neck. The patient receives a sedative and an anti-sickness drug and, if the lower half of the body is being treated, a drug to prevent diarrhoea. The treatment is given as one single large dose to the relevant part of the body and the patient remains in hospital overnight for observation. This form of treatment can be very effective, with dramatic resolution of pain and discomfort within twenty-four hours.

GENERAL ADVICE

- Ask questions of the radiographers and doctors you encounter during your treatment. Your relationship with medical staff is likely to be a long one, and misunderstandings may mean that it gets off on the wrong footing. Questions may not arise during the planning of the treatment, but in most centres there will be a weekly clinic where you will have the opportunity to discuss any problems.
- If a particular side effect seems severe, do not play it down. If the staff are not informed then appropriate investigations cannot be carried out and tablets prescribed to alleviate the symptoms.
- Be prepared to be adaptable and to take rests. It may be necessary to take time off work, to avoid frequent or prolonged breaks in treatment and to get plenty of rest. Having embarked on a course of radiotherapy, it is important that the time over which it is given is approximately the same as that which was intended. However, one day off to visit the palace for your knighthood would be perfectly acceptable to the doctor! Longer breaks may be unavoidable for personal reasons but if they can be anticipated it is worth mentioning them at the outset – it may even be preferable to start the treatment slightly later or to tailor the treatment to incorporate the outside commitment in some way.

SIDE EFFECTS OF RADIOTHERAPY

One side effect which many patients experience during their treatment is general fatigue and tiredness. This is to be expected, and you should not be at all surprised if you need an extra two to three hours' sleep per day. Otherwise, early side effects relate to the area being treated. If you are having a small area treated, particularly on the limbs, you are unlikely to experience much in the way of side effects. At worst, your skin may be slightly red and sore towards the end of the treatment (like a localised sunburn), but nausea, diarrhoea and lethargy are extremely unlikely. Only the area which is being treated is likely to be affected by the radiation. The exception to this is blood which continues to circulate during the treatment; consequently, any red or white blood cells which pass through the treatment area may well be damaged. This is of no significance in the majority of patients, but where a large area is being treated over a prolonged period of time, or the patient has had previous chemotherapy, the number of white blood cells, which fight infection, may be suppressed, increasing the risk of infection. Your doctor is likely to point out this problem during treatment and monitor your blood count more frequently.

Individuals vary in their sensitivity to radiation. The same dose may produce a severe skin reaction in one person and only a mild reaction in another. As a rule, the symptoms are worse towards the end of treatment and often reach a peak after four to five weeks. Nausea may be noticed at the beginning of treatment but gradually improves with time. This may be experienced when a large part of the body is treated. Nausea is particularly common during treatments to the abdomen although it may also be experienced by patients having treatment to nearby structures.

Side effects depend on the dose given, as well as on the size of the area being treated. With the advent of high-energy radiotherapy, treatment of a deep-seated tumour does not entail a particularly high dose to the skin and many patients in this category will have only a minimal skin reaction. Conversely, treatment to an area such as the breast does involve a reasonably large dose to the skin in order to control the size of the tumour, and here there may be quite marked soreness towards the end of the course. One of the most difficult regions for treatment is the head and neck area. In order to give a dose adequate to provide tumour control with minimal damage to tissue at a later stage, the treatment is likely to produce severe soreness of the mucous membranes inside the mouth and throat and, as a result, swallowing may become temporarily painful and difficult. Medication is readily available to help with these symptoms.

LONG-TERM SIDE EFFECTS

For each individual the significance of long-term side effects will vary. In young people, infertility may be a very high price to pay, whereas later in life, loss of hair may be the most demoralising aspect of treatment. It may be possible to overcome some of the long-term side effects in other ways: in a man, for example, infertility can be overcome by storing sperm. For a woman, the possibility of being left infertile may mean choosing between surgery or radiotherapy as the primary method of treatment. Again, you have every right to discuss the possible long-term effects with your doctor at the outset, so that you can decide together on the emphasis of your treatment and which side effects, if any, can be avoided. The benefits must be set against the price paid. Cure at any cost may not be justified. This may well be the case in an older patient, who feels that he has already lived a fulfilled and happy life.

Hair loss after radiotherapy is only a problem when the head itself has been treated. In the majority of patients it is not permanent and regrowth will start from as little as four to five weeks after treatment. If the patient has a slow-growing brain tumour, the dose to certain parts of the scalp may necessarily have been very high. This may result in permanent damage to some of the hair follicles and consequent thinning of the hair at a later stage. However, the advent of computer CT scanning and linear accelerators means that the scalp can often be spared, leaving the patient with a reasonably thick head of hair in the long term.

Only treatment of the pelvis will bring about infertility. This may be temporary. Treatment of one testis can be carried out with lead shielding the other testis, thereby preserving fertility. Treatment of pelvic tumours in women by means of radiotherapy may mean that surgery is not being used. In cervical cancer, surgery is used for early disease in younger women to conserve the ovaries (and avoid thickening of the skin of the vagina, making intercourse painful). Any woman who is considering having a child after treatment should consult her physician. Women on hormones or who have recently completed chemotherapy should avoid becoming pregnant.

A much more common late side effect, experienced in varying degrees, is the cosmetic result. A good illustration of this problem is the treatment of breast cancer after removal of the tumour. If the patient feels that the cosmetic result is not important to her, the treatment can be given in a small number of large doses with gaps between the treatments from a few days up to one week. The tumour control is comparable to that achieved using five- to six-week courses of radiotherapy. On the other hand, a treatment spread out over five to six weeks, giving small daily doses to the breast followed by an extra dose to the scar, is most likely to result in good control of the tumour and a soft breast. Many months after treatment it may be difficult to tell which breast has been treated. A number of methods can be used to give the extra treatment to the breast scar: these include electron beam therapy (a different type of radiotherapy, which treats only the 2–3 cm below the scar); a radioactive implant (which may be inserted under a general anaesthetic, after which the patient remains on the ward for a few days); or a reducing field technique, whereby the whole breast is treated initially and then the area of the breast in which the tumour is located is given a further dose. The cosmetic outcome of all these treatments is controversial – some physicians feel that top-up with a radioactive implant provides the best cosmetic result; others feel that electron beam therapy, given on an outpatient basis, is more convenient and does not entail the inevitable risk of a general anaesthetic. The long-term cosmetic results will become apparent over a period of months and years when the patient is followed up. Firmness in the breast, often particularly evident around the area of the scar where the top-up dose was given, may only be obvious one or two years after treatment, and may become more apparent over the subsequent years until it reaches a static point. For many patients this is not a major problem. The most important aspect is that when they go to the follow-up clinic they are reassured that this is a normal occurrence.

THE LIMITATIONS OF RADIOTHERAPY

Tumours are given a dose of radiotherapy which is close to the maximum tolerated by the normal tissues in this region. The risk of damage to normal tissue is the major factor limiting the use of radiotherapy and, for this reason, radiotherapy is only used to treat cancers which are localised (i.e. have not spread) at the time of treatment. Should the tumour recur, further radiotherapy would exceed the normal tissue tolerance and the patient might well suffer severe side effects – possibly fatal – from damage to such tissues. Sensitive structures include the brain, spinal cord, lungs, liver and bone marrow. It must be frustrating and sometimes incomprehensible when a tumour shrinks away after radiotherapy, but the same tumour cannot be dissipated a second time by the use of further radiotherapy.

Both radiotherapy and chemotherapy damage the source of rapidly dividing cells in the bone marrow and eventually the body may no longer be able to produce enough white blood cells, platelets and finally red blood cells. The amount of bone marrow treated by radiotherapy will subsequently limit the amount of chemotherapy which can be given for a particular disease. As a result of this restriction, no form of radiotherapy or chemotherapy should be given without seriously considering both the immediate effect and the long-term price to be paid.

MYTHS ABOUT RADIOTHERAPY

- *Do you lose your hair?*
  A common misconception is that radiotherapy inevitably causes hair loss. Radiotherapy can only cause hair loss if the scalp is within the area being treated. Similarly, axillary hair will be lost if the armpit is being treated but not otherwise.

- *Do you become radioactive?*

  A patient receiving radiotherapy from an external machine, which treats them at a distance from the body, is not radioactive. Those receiving implants of radioactive sources, either in the form of interstitial treatment (where radioactive wires are inserted into tissue such as the breast or tongue under anaesthetic) or a source within a body cavity, *will* become radioactive. But this is not as frightening as it sounds. The radiation is directed at the part of the body containing the tumour and is the best way of dealing with the problem. It does not hurt and has remarkably few side effects. There are very strict guidelines concerning the discharge of such patients from hospital if they are in any way likely to be radioactive. Consequently, radioactive sources are removed before the patient is discharged. Where this is not possible (where a radioactive liquid has been ingested), they are kept in hospital in a side room until the dose of radiation being emitted from the body is below the legal safe limit. Afterwards this dose continues to fall as the radioactive isotope decays.

- *Can you see X-rays?*

  You cannot see X- or gamma rays. The only visible part of the electromagnetic spectrum is the light we see. Radio, infra-red, ultra-violet, X- and gamma rays are all invisible. It is only their effects we witness.

- *Do you feel unwell during treatment?*

  It is a myth that all patients undergoing radiotherapy feel unwell, tired or nauseated. Many, particularly those having small areas treated, sail through therapy with only slight skin soreness and no other apparent side effects. Some patients benefit from treatment to such an extent that they feel much better at the end of treatment than they did at the beginning.

- *Can you take tablets or drugs during radiotherapy?*

  Within reason, no tablets or drugs are restricted during radiotherapy. Alcohol is discouraged in excess, particularly where the throat or oesophagus is being treated, and generally the intake of clear fluids is encouraged. It is important not to stop any regular medications suddenly and, if in doubt, it is best to ask the advice of your doctor or radiographers.

- *Can you wash during radiotherapy?*

    Contrary to what many patients may be told when they first attend for their treatment to be planned, you *can* wash during radiotherapy. The most important thing is to be sensible: the skin overlying the area which is being treated can be splashed with cold or lukewarm water, but it should not be scrubbed or rubbed dry and creams should be avoided. This is because towards the end of treatment the skin will become increasingly red and sore, and friction will make this problem worse. You should not use creams on your skin as this actually increases the dose of radiation to the skin surface and thereby makes the redness and burning worse. Once again, you should ask the radiographers' advice and alternative ways of relieving the symptoms may be suggested. One of the most upsetting aspects of treatment is the advice not to wash during therapy. This often restricts patients from having baths or showers completely unnecessarily, and a few well-directed questions can avoid all the misunderstanding. We even suggest to our patients that gentle shampooing of the head can be carried out weekly during treatment to this area.

HAVING RADIOTHERAPY PRIVATELY

The 'enterprise economy' mentality has engendered a feeling that by paying for treatment you are, in some way, obtaining a better service. There is very little to support this within the current NHS, particularly in relation to cancer care. Cancer is usually dealt with urgently, with patients being seen in the next available outpatient clinic, which very often is as soon as they would have been seen in the private sector.

The major advantages of private treatment are a personal room, better decor in the hospital, staff being slightly less harassed and the fact that you are likely to see the consultant at every visit. If you are fortunate enough to have a health care insurance policy which covers cancer treatment, then you should take advantage of it. However, if you have to pay for your treatment you may run out of money before your course of radiotherapy is finished. This unnecessary impoverishment limits resources for areas where money may make a significant difference.

Currently there are very few hospitals in Britain which provide radiotherapy entirely privately. Most private patients will be treated in NHS centres and the only fundamental difference in the treatment will be the medical staff who are dealing with them.

THE FACTORY PROBLEM

The cost of radiotherapy machinery and the number of staff involved in the treatment process mean that, with the exception of London, radiotherapy centres are relatively sparsely scattered around the country. You may need to travel long distances in order to receive an adequate service, and may be left with the feeling that you are simply another statistic. This may be very demoralising if you are coming to terms with a recent diagnosis of cancer. Some people find it possible to use this situation positively, deriving strength from the feeling of comradeship and mutual experience. The nurses, radiographers and doctors are another important resource which should be utilised in increasing individual understanding of the process of radiotherapy and its rationale. It is only through such insight that the fear and perceived lack of control, which might result from the disease and its treatment, can be avoided.

FOLLOW-UP VISITS

Once the initial radical treatment has been completed, you will visit the hospital regularly as an outpatient so that your consultant can check whether your skin, which looks very sunburnt after treatment, has returned to normal and, where possible, to assess your response to treatment. In many cancers this takes the form of a 'wait and see' approach. You may have had investigations before and during radiotherapy to assess the extent of your disease. These may include X-rays, scans and blood tests. At this point, the important distinction for both you and your doctor is whether the disease is confined to the primary site, or has spread outside this region. There is no guarantee in any patient that there are not microscopic clumps of cancer cells outside the primary site for unless these are at least 5 mm in diameter they will not be detectable with any of the currently available technology.

Initially your follow-up visits will be relatively frequent – probably every two to three months. As time goes by, these visits will become more spread out and may be six months or even a year apart. The period of follow-up is variable and there are no hard-and-fast rules. If you find outpatient attendances upsetting and feel that you can take responsibility for noting symptoms, or detecting any changes, then it may be reasonable for clinic visits to be kept to a minimum – with the proviso that you reattend the clinic if you feel in any way worried about new developments. Many cancers carry a 99 per cent chance of having been cured if no symptoms have recurred after five years. This is particularly true of most head and neck cancers, lung cancers and some sarcomas. However, most patients are followed up for about ten years. With diseases such as the lymphomas, there is a small risk of second malignancy. For this reason, most lymphoma patients are followed up for life. Breast cancer is in a different category, and even twenty years after the primary treatment it is not unknown for a patient to develop secondary deposits. Such very late recurrences often respond well to hormone therapy and it may be feasible to prolong a patient's life for many years.

An annual visit to the clinic, or an understanding that you can return promptly with any worries, means that such recurrences can be detected early and consequently are more likely to be curable. The follow-up clinic is a useful time to ask any questions, to express any fears and to seek reassurance about any late side effects which may have arisen. Without an explanation from the doctor at such a time, these problems, particularly unexpected, might otherwise prove very alarming.

CASE HISTORY

Miss H was a medical student who at the age of twenty noticed a sore on the roof of her mouth. A sample of tissue revealed a melanoma (that is, a tumour arising from the pigmented cells in the skin). There was a hole at the centre of the sore which connected with the cavity at the back of the nose. Treatment was carried out with radiotherapy from six different directions. Two directions were treated at any one time, so that the normal tissue was spared as much as possible. During treatment the hole closed up, the sore healed and apart from minimal soreness of the roof of the mouth, there were virtually no side effects. Within four weeks of treatment the redness had resolved completely and only a small indentation was visible. Some years later she had no further problems in spite of the usual very poor prognosis. More importantly, extensive disfiguring surgery had been completely avoided. This case history shows how radiotherapy can sometimes have an advantage over surgery. It also demonstrates that with the technological advances of the last decade the side effects of radiotherapy are not what they were and it is not a form of treatment to be feared.

CHEMOTHERAPY

We have seen in the previous chapters how cancer can be treated effectively by surgery or radiotherapy when it is localised to a defined site in the body. But the main problem with cancer is that it spreads – firstly, along the lymphatic channels to local lymph nodes and then on into the bloodstream and beyond into other organs. Surgery and radiotherapy can only deal with local disease. When spread has taken place, the treatment which has to be given must be **systemic**. That means it has to go right round the body, following the cancer cells in their trail of destruction.

Until 1944, there was no known drug effective against cancer. At the end of the Second World War, the US military began experimenting with new chemical weapons. They stumbled upon the alkylating agents – drugs that bind to the DNA, the thread of life present in every cell. Basically these agents completely destroy the mechanism by which DNA produces its message. The first of these agents was nitrogen mustard, and there were many other related compounds. During field trials in which volunteer soldiers were exposed to the alkylating agents during military manoeuvres, it was found that the white cell count in the blood fell dramatically. This prompted Louis Goodman, an American pharmacologist, to use one of the alkylating agents in a patient with lymphoma. (A lymphoma is a tumour of the lymph nodes.) Goodman's patient also had a raised white blood count caused by tumour cells spilling into the blood. To everyone's amazement, the blood count fell and the patient's enlarged lymph node shrank rapidly after just one injection of mustine. The drug had unpleasant side effects, causing very severe nausea and vomiting shortly after its administration. But shrinkage of the tumour was dramatic. Several patients went through this new treatment for cancer amid great excitement. But then it was noted that many patients did not actually respond. Only those with lymphomas and leukaemias had dramatic improvements in their condition. Even here the disease started to grow again in between courses of mustine. Patients could only tolerate the drug in small amounts as it was found to be very poisonous to their normal bone marrow, resulting in abnormal bleeding. It also suppressed the patient's innate defence mechanisms against bacteria, leading to an increased risk of infection.

But although the initial optimism was unfounded, a breakthrough had been made: a systemic drug was available for the treatment of cancer. Since 1945, around 100 drugs with anti-cancer effects have been discovered. Some are useful in several types of cancer, whereas others are very specific in the tumours they can control. Some drugs work at the level of DNA, preventing it from being copied – a vital process in cell division. These drugs bind directly to DNA itself, distorting its structure and preventing the attachment of the enzymes necessary for it to divide and reproduce. Other drugs deplete the cell of the building blocks for DNA so that fewer raw materials are available for DNA replication. Still other drugs prevent binding of the enzymes to produce RNA, the message of the thread of life, vital in the production of proteins – the executive molecules of the cell. Drugs have been devised that block protein synthesis, essential for the maintenance of cell activity and also for its division. The periwinkle plant produces a family of drugs, collectively known as the vinca-alkaloids, which block cell division by preventing the small bundles of intra-cellular muscles from pulling chromosomes apart at the time of cell division.

THE DISCOVERY OF ANTI-CANCER DRUGS

The majority of the anti-cancer drugs that we use were discovered by accident. Few were designed specifically to inhibit tumour cell growth.

During the 1950s the National Cancer Institute in Washington, which is the largest cancer research enterprise in the world, embarked on a very ambitious testing programme with a whole range of substances. Scientists collected chemicals from all over the world from all sorts of sources, and tested them for their ability to kill cancer cells. This programme uncovered a variety of structures which we still use to this day. Over a million compounds have now been screened and vast banks of data collected by this process have been accumulated in the archives of the National Cancer Institute.

There are more romantic stories about the discovery of anti-cancer drugs. Several pharmaceutical companies developed programmes to search for new drugs in fungi and algae, looking for a repeat of the famous penicillin story of Alexander Fleming. High above the Adriatic Sea, in northern Italy, is an old tower built in mediaeval times. The tower itself is a crumbling ruin overgrown with moss and ivy. Samples of fungus were taken from this beautiful tower and from these a drug that inserted itself within the stacked base pairs of DNA was identified. This drug was remarkably effective in controlling breast cancer, non-Hodgkin's lymphoma and many other tumour types. It was named adriamycin, as it had been discovered on the Adriatic coast.

The discovery of cisplatinum, commonly used for testicular cancer, sarcomas and gynaecological tumours, is another interesting story. In the early 1960s an American scientist, Bill Rosenberg, was interested in the ability of electric fields to inhibit bacterial growth. He was a pure scientist working in the laboratory with no intent of developing new anti-cancer agents. His experimental system was relatively simple. He grew bacteria in a small dish and measured how many would grow in a defined period of time. He then inserted two electrodes and passed an electric current between them. He noticed that the growth rate of the bacteria diminished when the electric current was switched on. Initially, he came to the conclusion that the electric current inhibited bacterial cell growth. Being of an enquiring mind, he performed the following experiment. He took fluid from bacteria which had been inhibited by the passage of an electric current and added it to fresh bacteria. Much to his surprise, he found that the growth rate of the second lot of bacteria was also diminished, even though no electric current had been passed through. A substance was produced by the passage of electric current that inhibited cell growth. This substance was found to be soluble platinum, produced by the passage of electricity through the platinum electrodes used in the experiment. Platinum is a precious metal used for jewellery and several industrial purposes. Although familiar as a shiny, silvery metallic solid, its organic form is a white, crystalline powder. Cisplatinum was the first of a series of platinum-containing complexes which were found to have considerable effect on certain tumours. A chance observation had given rise to a new group of anti-cancer drugs.

The initial discovery of alkylating agents led to the screening of many other drugs that would bind to DNA. Some drugs were designed to increase their solubility or their ability to concentrate in tumours. Drugs have also been modified to try and reduce side effects. Cisplatinum, for example, has very profound effects on the kidney. It causes irreversible damage to the small tubes of the kidney with subsequent kidney failure. To avoid this, patients are given a large amount of fluid by intravenous infusion prior to the administration of cisplatinum. This means that patients usually have to come into hospital. A drug with a similar structure, carboplatin, has been designed and this is less damaging to the kidneys and avoids the need for hospital admission. Unfortunately, carboplatin has more bone marrow damage potential.

SIDE EFFECTS

Because tumour cells are so close in structure and function to normal cells, it is not surprising that any drug that reduces cancer growth also affects normal cells. This means that many drugs have very potent side effects. For this reason they are usually prescribed only by specialists in the field. Thus, GPs and other hospital doctors do not get involved in cancer drug administration as it can be a lethal process unless in skilled hands. Anti-cancer drugs inhibit cell turnover generally and so, not surprisingly, it is the most rapidly dividing cells in the body – the bone marrow, lining of the intestine, skin and hair follicles – that can be most severely affected.

In the skin, itching can occur and hair loss is common. Some drugs are more notorious for causing hair loss than others. Adriamycin is particularly bad. Although attempts have been made to reduce hair loss by putting elastic bands round the scalp or cooling the hair, none of these methods is effective in the long term. Depression of the bone marrow results in decline of the red cells (leading to anaemia), the white cells (leading to a decrease in leucocytes and depressed defences against infection), and thrombocytopenia when the platelets (tiny factors vital for blood clotting) are depleted. Anaemia can easily be corrected by blood transfusion; but thrombocytopenia can result in abnormal bleeding into body cavities, or to the exterior. To avoid problems of bone marrow depression, patients having chemotherapy have a blood test to check their blood count and kidney function every time chemotherapy is given. The dose and number of drugs given can then be adjusted if necessary. Some drugs cause the cells lining the intestine to switch off, leading to severe diarrhoea and fluid loss. Suppression of the immune system is common with many anti-cancer drugs. This decreases the defence against infection and patients may be more susceptible to sore throats and other unpleasant symptoms. Patients having chemotherapy are regularly checked by their physicians looking for infection. Any signs of it are dealt with rapidly by using appropriate antibiotics.

Another curious effect of many anti-cancer drugs is that they can cause specific changes in single organs. For example, adriamycin in large quantities is toxic to the muscle of the heart, resulting in circulatory problems in a few patients. Similarly, bleomycin causes fibrosis in the lung. This can cause shortness of breath or shadows on a chest X-ray. Cisplatinum can cause kidney damage. Several other drugs result in skin pigmentation. It is for this reason that some patients on long term anti-cancer drugs may look darker than normal.

Part of good cancer management is trying to administer drugs, and combinations of drugs, in such a way as to maximise their effect on the tumour and minimise their effect on normal cells. The best way to do this is to give the drugs in large doses, at intervals of three to four weeks. This allows the normal bone marrow to recover in between. Tumour cells are not so well able to repair the damage caused by the drugs as their normal counterparts. One of the major problems in the treatment of certain cancers is drug resistance. It is thought that giving several drugs together in large doses will kill tumour cells before they have a chance to develop resistance.

One side effect that is often neglected is the psychological impact on a patient and his family of repeated hospital visits, often with a lot of waiting around for blood count results and, in some cases, unpleasant nausea and vomiting. The latter are caused by the effect of chemotherapy directly on the lining of the stomach and on a zone at the back of the brain. This zone is responsible for sea sickness. Certain types of irregular swinging motion cause signals to be sent from the inner ear to this zone, inducing sickness in some patients. This varies tremendously from patient to patient. Some drugs may cause severe vomiting in one patient and not affect another. Thankfully, there is a variety of drugs now available that block vomiting. These can increase stomach emptying, suppress the vomiting centre directly and confuse the brain into thinking all is well. Perhaps the most interesting is a drug called nabilone. This is a synthetic derivative of cannabis or marijuana. It was noted in hippy days of the 1960s in California, that patients who smoked pot weren't sick during chemotherapy. Those who did not smoke would take 'hash-brownies'. Hash-brownies are little brown chocolate cakes into which marijuana is mixed before baking. Some patients liked the mild hallucinogenic effect and the dream-like trance which seemed to stop the sickness caused by the chemotherapy. Nabilone is synthetic – made in the chemistry laboratory. It is similar to marijuana, but does not cause hallucinations.

If a patient gets severe vomiting with chemotherapy, he needs to be given anti-sickness drugs before actually going to hospital to have chemotherapy. The story of Pavlov's dogs and conditioned reflexes explains why. Pavlov, a pioneering Russian psychologist, studied salivation in dogs. He noted that when dogs were given meat they would salivate and drool if they were hungry. He rang a bell just before giving the meat. After a period of time, the dogs learnt to salivate on hearing the bell even if they were not given the meat. This process is called **conditioning**. We are all subject to conditioning from the day we are born. Vomiting when undergoing chemotherapy is a similar response: if a patient is violently sick the first time he has chemotherapy, then he tends to associate the two; he *expects* to be sick and so he is. If this first unpleasant experience of vomiting can be prevented, then serious vomiting is less likely to take place later. In extreme cases, a patient can actually start to feel sick when he sees anything associated with his chemotherapy. This may be watching a film about hospital life on television, or even more bizarre, when he sees his doctor at the supermarket on a Saturday morning. But there are now more powerful anti-nausea drugs so, hopefully, conditioning will be a thing of the past.

HOW ANTI-CANCER DRUGS ARE GIVEN

There are many ways in which drugs can be taken into the body and, of course, this applies to those against cancer. Some can be taken as pills or capsules. Unfortunately, many anti-cancer drugs are complex and would be damaged inside the stomach or intestine, or broken down along with the food we eat. For this reason, many are given by injection into a vein. Some, such as mustine and adriamycin, cause tissue breakdown when concentrated. To prevent this they are diluted by running the drug into a fast-flowing drip so that it is carried away in the bloodstream, being diluted as it goes. To reduce the side effects some drugs are diluted in a bottle, or bag, of fluid which is hung up as a drip leading into a vein.

Most anti-cancer drugs can be given in the outpatient clinic. The patient arrives, a blood sample is taken for the blood count to be determined and the patient seen by a doctor to check that all is well. When the blood count result arrives, the doctor writes the prescription for the course of chemotherapy which is then obtained from pharmacy. Some combinations of drugs use a mixture of tablet and injection. These combinations have been found by trial and error to be the best for that particular disease. Here are some examples of drug combinations producing cures.

Lymphomas

Lymphomas consist of Hodgkin's disease (about 40 per cent) and non-Hodgkin's lymphoma (60 per cent). The latter are broadly divided into low-grade and high-grade tumours. Low-grade tumours are just that: they cause symptoms from time to time and these tend to respond to mild treatment, often in tablet form. High-grade tumours used to be fatal, but using similar drug combinations to those used in Hodgkin's disease a proportion have now been cured.

Hodgkin's disease

Until 1965 the majority of patients with this disease died. Only those whose tumour was localised to a small area that could be effectively irradiated were cured. Hodgkin's disease is a lymphoma – a cancer of the cells that make up the lymphatic system. These lymphocytes are part of the blood's white cell complement and vital for defence against bacteria and viruses. Doctors tried using new anti-cancer drugs in patients with this lymphoma as soon as they became available in the mid-1940s. Although the drugs significantly reduced the amount of tumour present they did not eradicate it completely. Then in 1965 the National Cancer Institute in Washington decided to treat patients with four drugs simultaneously. Each drug was known to be of some help individually, and they hoped that their combined effects would produce a cure.

These four drugs – mustine, vincristine, procarbazine and prednisolone – were given over a fortnight. Two were given as tablets every day, and the others by injection on the first and eighth day. Called MOPP after the initial letters of the four drugs (the trade name for vincristine is Oncovin), the combination resulted in the complete and permanent disappearance of Hodgkin's disease from many patients. Many of those who received MOPP in 1965 are still alive today. Oncologists still use a very similar combination of drugs for the treatment of Hodgkin's disease.

This was a dramatic breakthrough. It led to new approaches in combining existing drugs for a whole range of different cancer types. Over the next decade, four different types of cancer became curable in many patients: lymphoma, testicular cancer, choriocarcinoma and childhood leukaemia.

Childhood leukaemia

More than 70 per cent of children with cancer can now be cured using a combination of surgery, radiotherapy and chemotherapy. The commonest, and most curable, childhood cancer is leukaemia.

Initially all leukaemia patients are **induced** – they have intensive treatment over two to three weeks, using four or five different drugs. At the end of this time 95 per cent of the children have no evidence of leukaemia in their blood or bone marrow. After an interval, during which the normal blood cells can recover, the treatment may be **consolidated** with a further intensive programme of chemotherapy. Patients with a particularly poor outlook may have two periods of consolidation. Because many of the chemotherapy drugs do not cross into the fluid around the brain and spinal cord, patients also undergo radiotherapy to those areas to make sure than any leukaemia cells which may be in the fluid are destroyed.

After completing this intensive period, the children then receive maintenance therapy – one drug on a daily basis, another weekly and a monthly injection. The period of maintenance therapy is currently two years.

Testicular cancer

Until 1975 there was little chance that patients with widespread testicular cancer could be treated with chemotherapy. The response to single drugs was not good and lasted for only a short time. The combination of three drugs – cisplatinum, vinblastine and bleomycin – dramatically increased the response rate. Over the subsequent years the regimen has been modified to reduce toxicity whilst retaining the high success rate. The most frequently used combination is now BEP – bleomycin, etoposide and cisplatinum. Studies are in progress to see whether the number, and duration, of courses or the doses of drugs can be reduced in those patients with the best outlook. In the majority of patients with testicular cancer the response can be monitored in a precise way, by measurement of marker proteins shed by the tumour into the serum.

In order to receive BEP the patient is admitted to hospital. A drip is put up and three litres of fluid are passed through it every day for five days, in addition to the fluids drunk. This promotes the flow of water through the kidneys protecting them from the toxic effects of cisplatinum. A careful watch is kept on fluid balance. If the patient is sick, then any lost fluid is made up by increasing the volume given in the drip that day. Cisplatinum is given in five daily divided doses into the vein, as is the etoposide. The bleomycin is given intravenously as a single injection every course. Three weeks after day one the patient returns for a further course, provided that the blood count and tests of kidney function are normal. In most patients four such cycles are enough to produce a cure.

Choriocarcinoma

This is a very rare tumour which arises from cells of the placenta. The symptoms usually develop during pregnancy with severe nausea and vomiting. Choriocarcinoma is sensitive to a similar combination of drugs to testicular cancer. Both arise from cells involved in reproduction known as germ cells, and are sensitive to the same chemotherapy agents.

SOME COMMON ANTI-CANCER DRUGS

Drug	Type of cancer	How given
adriamycin	breast, lung, sarcomas	intravenously
bleomycin	testicular, lymphoma	intravenously
	head and neck tumours	intramuscularly
cisplatinum	ovary, testicular, lung	intravenously
chlorambucil	ovary, leukaemia, lymphoma	orally
cyclophosphamide	breast, lymphoma	orally or intravenously

5-fluorouracil	colon, stomach, pancreas	orally or intravenously
methotrexate	bladder, breast, lung	orally or intravenously
vincristine	lymphoma, childhood tumours, kidney, brain	intravenously

DRUG RESISTANCE

Drug resistance is perhaps the biggest problem in chemotherapy today. Although there has been great success in some cancer types, many common tumours are difficult to cure. It sometimes seems to be part of the behaviour pattern of a tumour right from the start. For this reason certain types of lung cancer are difficult to treat. Breast and ovarian cancer respond readily to existing drugs, but become resistant within six months to one year in most cases. In some patients there is drug resistance at the onset. Often the cells are resistant to a number of drugs. On the plus side there are some cancers, such as testicular cancer and Hodgkin's disease, which are not resistant at the start and rarely develop problems, just melting away with successive courses, in a predictable fashion.

Tumour cells are rather clever. They can adapt to unfavourable surroundings. They do this by increasing their ability to destroy anti-cancer drugs by producing more of the enzyme required for their breakdown. Alternatively, they may develop special mechanisms to increase the export of, not just one, but several anti-cancer drugs at the same time. There is a molecule which actively pumps a number of drugs out of the cell. This sits astride the cell membrane. Tumour cells with large quantities of this molecule have evolved and so show a survival advantage over those tumour cells without it. The tumour is soon made up of cells with an increased amount of export protein, and so becomes drug-resistant. Over the last few years, doctors have gained considerable insight into the molecular mechanisms of drug resistance and, hopefully, will soon be able to combat it.

Hormonal Therapy

Hormonal therapy, using substances normally produced by the body, can also be used to treat certain cancers. Hormones are chemical messengers produced by the endocrine glands. These include the pituitary at the base of the brain, the thyroid in the neck, the adrenals above the kidneys and the ovaries in women and testes in men. Many hormones control the normal growth of specific tissues. For example, the female sex hormone oestrogen is produced in the ovary and stimulates the growth of cells in the breast.

In 1896, George Beatson, a Scottish surgeon, removed the ovaries of two young patients with advanced breast cancer. In both women the disease stopped growing and regressed. Though the tumours later returned, this was the first demonstration that changing the circulating levels of hormones could be effective against cancer. We now know that the removal of the ovaries leads to a fall in levels of oestrogen in the blood. The amount of oestrogen reaching the breast tumour is therefore less and the rate of tumour growth is reduced. Since then hormonal therapy has been widely used for cancers arising in tissues susceptible to hormonal influences such as the breast, prostate and uterus.

There are three ways that the level of hormone activity can be influenced. The first is to destroy the endocrine gland that produces it by surgery, radiotherapy or drugs. The second approach is to give a hormone. Paradoxically, using very large doses of some natural hormones to overwhelm the tissue which has developed cancer inhibits the cancer cells. Patients with breast cancer may consequently receive extra oestrogen. Alternatively, the hormone given may be one that the body would not normally secrete. Prostate cancer in men is often treated with oestrogen as this female hormone inhibits the growth of prostate tissue. The third technique is to develop drugs that block the effects of a hormone. For hormones to work they have to interact with receptors in their target tissue. This can be likened to a key (the hormone) fitting a lock (the receptor). If another substance fits the same lock but does not activate it, the hormone's effect can be blocked. Such drugs are called anti-hormones. The best example is tamoxifen, which blocks the action of oestrogen and is often used in treating breast cancer.

But not all patients respond to hormonal treatment. Responses may be variable even in cancers arising in the same tissue. Hormone treatment has relatively few side effects. There is no bone marrow depression or hair loss. For this reason hormones are often used as the main form of therapy in those tumours likely to be responsive.

MEDICAL ONCOLOGY

Medical oncology is the name given to the speciality involving the administration of anti-cancer drugs. Most doctors are not experienced in the use of these drugs. Indeed, many can only be prescribed in specialist units. Different countries have evolved different strategies of how to administer them. In the UK a network of cancer centres of varying size is responsible for the care of most patients. Most chemotherapy is given by doctors who give both radiotherapy and chemotherapy. Their title is Consultant in Radiotherapy and Oncology. There are around 250 in the country. Medical oncology is a much smaller speciality, with only about fifty consultants. In many centres, radiotherapists and medical oncologists work very closely together with surgeons and others to make sure the cancer treatment planned for an individual is the best possible. But, there is still the odd lone wolf who may not be up to date in all aspects of modern cancer care. Treatment in a larger centre is usually preferable because the pool of expertise is greater. Even though it may be inconvenient to travel to another town for treatment, it is often worthwhile. Many specialists visit hospitals in surrounding districts to try to reduce travelling by the patient. They may even give chemotherapy in small hospitals.

The danger comes when a specialist fails to realise that he is no longer in touch with modern trends in the treatment of a specific condition. This can happen at a time of change for the better in the results of treating a particular tumour type. A good example is the widely differing results obtained in different centres in the UK for the treatment of testicular cancer between 1982 and 1985. Some five years previously, the Americans had pioneered chemotherapy programmes containing platinum, and these should have been generally available within the UK. But the level of expertise varied enormously. During those years the mortality from testicular cancer at five centres, all within 100 miles radius of each other, was compared. The centres treating more patients were clearly getting better results. This is because they had the concentration of expertise to deal with particular clinical problems, and were more aware of developments on a worldwide basis.

Another area where concentration of expertise is essential is children's cancer. Fortunately, cancer is rare in children and also amenable to expert treatment. But treatment is often complicated and needs the resources of a group of specialists dealing with a whole range of child care problems. Treating an occasional child with leukaemia by looking in a textbook and copying out a drug regimen is a recipe for disaster. It is only by the concentration of resources and patients at centres of excellence that optimal care can be assured. This is vital for tumours that are potentially curable.

GETTING THE RIGHT TREATMENT

If you do not take responsibility for this, why should anybody else? You are quite entitled to know exactly what plans doctors have for your treatment in hospital. This book should help you to understand the problems in treating cancer. A discussion with your own GP should help put it in the right perspective. But at the end of the day, it is the responsibility of those giving chemotherapy to explain how it will be done, the side effects it might cause and its potential benefit. Nearly all involved, whether nurses or doctors, will be happy to explain things that seem unclear. Some patients are afraid to ask for fear of seeming stupid. Don't be. Always ask until you are satisfied that you have enough information.

If you are still in doubt you can seek a second opinion. As for surgery and radiotherapy, it is vital that the consultant giving the second opinion has all your medical details and the proposed plan in front of him, otherwise he cannot come to any rational decision. For this reason, your GP should send a note detailing the situation together with the results of any investigations. In this way, a single consultation can be extremely useful. Second opinions are freely available under the NHS and also privately.

Private chemotherapy

Having chemotherapy privately, confers no advantage over getting it in the NHS. If you are paying your own way, the drugs are often very expensive, up to £1200 a course. The advantage is that you will be seen by the consultant more regularly, but the drawbacks are that you only have the benefit of his advice and not the other doctors that form part of the team. Furthermore, if problems arise, and the consultant is not available, there will be no one else familiar with your case. There may well be less waiting time and the surroundings may be more pleasant. But the drugs themselves, the way they are given, and their chances of success are exactly the same.

CLINICAL TRIALS

Clinical trials are necessary to determine whether new drugs are effective or whether, when offered in combination, they have fewer side effects with the same potential for destroying tumours. Clinical trials are an essential part of modern anti-cancer treatment. It's only by doing such studies that things can improve. You may well be asked to join in a clinical trial. It is purely voluntary, and of course there is no obligation. A consent form will require your signature and a full explanation of the study will be given. You should use this opportunity to ask anything else about your disease that worries you.

All clinical trials have to be approved by a hospital ethics committee, consisting of doctors and lay people. This considers a wide range of ethical issues about the study. Above all, an ethics committee will decide whether the new treatment proposed is likely to be as effective as existing treatment. If this is not confirmed by the results, there is a failsafe system for stopping the trial at any point and switching to conventional treatment. As well as contributing to future knowledge, participating in a clinical trial can bring other dividends. You will be more closely monitored and perhaps have more frequent checks on your health and well-being than if not on a study. Most objections from patients come because of misunderstandings. It is your body, so make sure you know exactly what is being tried and why. Not only you but many others may benefit as a result of your taking part.

COMPLEMENTARY MEDICINE

Being told you have cancer is a traumatic and isolating experience, no matter how hard your doctor tries to soften the blow. Medical teaching in the past two decades has attempted to raise doctors' awareness of this, but shortage of time and a hospital setting don't make things any easier. Many patients with cancer will die from it and this is not something that anyone can accept lightly. Virtually half of all patients experience psychological and emotional problems and this may well be a conservative estimate. Obtaining support at the outset, in the form of information and counselling, may prevent much of this stress. Increasing numbers of cancer treatment departments recognise the need for psychological support and employ counsellors or psychotherapists, with formal training in this area, to help both inpatients and outpatients. Seeking help from a psychologist at such a difficult time is certainly not something to be ashamed of. In addition, there are many self-help groups, help lines and cancer support centres. Most of these have no formal link with the NHS and are self-funded.

WHAT IS COMPLEMENTARY MEDICINE?

Complementary medicine is just that – an attempt to complement, and not thwart, conventional care. Complementary medicine concentrates on the whole person, rather than just on the disease, and is based on the belief that your attitudes and state of mind have a great influence on your physical health: if you are happy, relaxed and optimistic then your physical health is likely to be better than if you are miserable and depressed. This approach to medicine is often used to treat diseases where health and resistance to infection are keys to recovery. Cancer is one such disease. Great emphasis is placed on self-healing and the wide range of therapies available is usually harmless. Most forms of complementary medicine start by looking at your lifestyle in general to see if there are any fears or psychological problems which might have a bearing on your present state. Of course, this does not mean that everyone with cancer has psychological problems which must be treated; but complementary medicine believes that for your body to be healthy and able to fight any disease, your mind must also be healthy.

The atmosphere of a hospital is often very high-tech and impersonal and many people find that this increases their anxiety. The result is that they find it hard to communicate with the staff around them and may bottle up their emotions until they are back in a familiar, comfortable atmosphere. This is where complementary medicine may come in. The problem with complementary medicine is that it is often difficult to find out what's available, the skills of its practitioners and how much it will cost. Other than counselling, there is little currently available on the NHS.

One place where help is readily available is the Cancer Help Centre at Bristol, which has pioneered a well-organised approach that many have found very helpful. The Centre offers either day- or week-long residential courses for patients and their carers. At the start of the week counselling sessions with doctors and nurses help to identify the type of treatment programme likely to be most beneficial. All sorts of complementary therapies, from special diets to healing, can be explored to find which best suits an individual's needs. Group sessions allow common problems to be shared so that a patient no longer feels so isolated. An atmosphere of peace pervades the Centre, quite unlike most hospital wards or clinics. At the end of the week, day sessions are arranged so that the lessons learnt can be reinforced. Many find themselves better able to cope with orthodox treatment after this experience. The current cost of a day at Bristol is around

£80 with the week-long residential programme costing £500. This is very good value compared to conventional private medicine. Bursaries are available to help with payment. We strongly recommend this organised approach rather than just seeing the first local counsellor advised by a well-meaning friend. There is a world of difference between Bristol and the sort of people advertising their services as hypnotists, nutrition experts and so on.

Complementary medicine – what is available

- counselling
- acupuncture
- homeopathy
- herbalism
- meditation and yoga
- visualisation
- relaxation
- massage
- osteopathy
- hypnotherapy
- dietary treatments

DIFFERENT PATIENTS' VIEWS

If you feel you would like to explore other methods of treatment in addition to conventional medicine, you must voice your needs, and ask about the complementary medicine available – that within the hospital itself, in the locality and on a national basis. The response you obtain is likely to vary from one consultant to another, but doctors are coming to recognise that patients have widely differing needs. Counselling in a hospital setting is becoming increasingly available. Complementary medicine may be a helpful way of coming to terms with the diagnosis of cancer and getting through conventional treatment. No two patients react in the same way to the diagnosis, and so their approach to treatment and their ability to carry on with their lives afterwards will also differ. Some want to abdicate responsibility to their specialist, others want to feel completely in control and therefore need as much information about their disease and its management as possible. Others have fixed ideas about their disease and its likely outcome, which no amount of persuasion can dislodge. Just as everyone will have a different approach to their illness, the help and information provided must be tailored to meet their individual requirements.

THE EXTREMISTS

A proportion of doctors within the NHS will be cynical about the use of complementary medicine but, by the same token, some complementary medicine practitioners will pour scorn on conventional treatment. This may undermine your confidence in the treatment you have had or are likely to be offered in the future. Both extremes are unhelpful for patient and doctor alike – providing one form of treatment does not compromise the effectiveness of the other – and it is best to be open-minded. For example, a patient receiving abdominal radiotherapy might insist on religiously adhering to a strict vegan diet, which contains no meat, eggs, milk or cheese. The high intake of largely raw food contains much roughage and is likely to stimulate the bowel, so making the side effects of abdominal radiotherapy worse. There must be a middle ground between these two approaches.

COUNSELLING

Consulting a counsellor is not simply a question of being told how to cope with cancer and being led along a straightforward path which contains all the answers. It is often about admitting that you need help and using the counsellor as a means of finding out how you can help yourself. There is a British 'stiff upper lip' resistance to obtaining psychological support which stems from a belief that people should be able to sort their problems out for themselves. Simply expressing your fears and anxieties may make it easier for you to cope with your feelings. A trouble shared is very often a trouble halved. After you have overcome your initial reluctance, it is possible to work through the feelings, obtaining some solace from what might otherwise be a very painful situation.

Counselling may be necessary not only to discuss the situation that has arisen and its implications, but also to view life more objectively, assess your own reaction to the situation and the contribution which this itself makes. It is not uncommon for families experiencing such intense emotions to vent them by expressing anger or resentment towards another individual – possibly a member of the family or a friend.

There are no hard and fast rules as to who should be a counsellor. Many NHS departments employ one. Cancer charities and a large proportion of complementary medicine centres will be able to advise, if not offer their own counsellor. A professional counsellor has probably had formal training over a period of months or years and will have experience of cancer sufferers and their families. However, a GP, or another partner in the same surgery who has experience in counselling and psychotherapy, may provide a preferable alternative for many individuals as they can be approached more discreetly and anonymously. Accepting that there is a problem and asking for help is more than half the battle. Once you can look the problem directly in the face, you are in a position to do something about it. A counsellor is simply acting as a catalyst to expedite the process.

Sometimes people who have experienced the death of a close friend or relative, or have suffered from cancer themselves, subsequently find a sense of purpose in their lives by becoming counsellors and setting up support groups which make things that much easier for other people. Dr Vicky Clement-Jones, a doctor at St Bartholomew's, was one such person. Having had ovarian cancer, she felt there was a need for an organisation such as BACUP (British Association of Cancer United Patients). This organisation, operating from the heart of London, provides free telephone advice to cancer patients and families. It is staffed by specially trained nurses who are able to give specific information about different cancer types and on services available locally. It now receives over 100 calls a day from all over the

UK. When it first started many doctors were sceptical and some even opposed it, feeling that it might undermine patients' confidence. But now most doctors realise how useful such a service can be and some hospitals are trying to provide their own cancer information units for patients. There is now a freephone line for people telephoning from outside London.

As well as individual counselling, joining a self-help group may well be useful. Here a group of patients meet, usually with a group leader, to discuss their feelings. Many find this helpful but a few dread going along. Our advice is not to be bullied by well-meaning relatives or friends to do anything you feel uncomfortable about. Information about such groups should be available at the hospital involved in your treatment – if not, telephone BACUP for details.

There are also a number of smaller more specific societies with interest in particular malignancies which have been founded by the relatives of victims of the disease, and have provided support that did not exist when they were faced with a similar situation.

RELAXATION

There are numerous forms of relaxation and meditation which can be used to help cancer patients and their families. Many people cope with periods of severe emotional stress by phrenetic over-activity. They become absorbed in some alternative pastime in the hope that they can shut out their emotions until much of the pain has passed. Relaxation and meditation provide a means to a positive mental attitude. This is something which is always to be encouraged both by those involved with conventional treatment of cancer and those concerned with complementary therapy. Such a positive attitude makes treatment more tolerable, is likely to improve the patient's general well-being and logically should improve the individual's chance of being one of those one in one hundred thousand people whose malignancy spontaneously regresses.

There are some extreme views for which there is little scientific evidence. Lawrence LeShan believes that cancer can be conquered by suppressing the 'cancer personality' – the very attributes which led to the person developing cancer in the first place. LeShan believes that, 'the people most capable of recovery are those who can discover a new well spring of hope and move on to a fresh sense of themselves, a true recognition of their worth as human beings'. This is perfectly acceptable if your malignancy is likely to be curable or you are in the small proportion who have a spontaneous remission.

Unfortunately for many patients, such an approach may well result in guilt on the part of the victim or blame of their families and loved ones for providing an environment in which cancer was able to develop. The diagnosis of cancer can carry with it enough feelings of blame and guilt under normal circumstances, without having to search for hidden psychological clues as to what caused it. There is a danger in suggesting that cancer is the result of stress, since modern life, for many reasons, is more likely to be stressful. People who smoke, eat unwisely and spend long periods in the sun are more likely to develop cancer than teetotal, non-smoking workaholics. With that proviso, it is nevertheless sensible to accept that cancer is an enormous challenge and that in order to meet that challenge it is appropriate to dissipate the effects of emotional stress through relaxation and meditation.

Meditation is a state of freedom from thought and in this respect is comparable to sleep. In the process physical activity and therefore the body's metabolic rate are decreased and it has a restoring quality which, for those who are able to meditate, is generally more versatile than sleep! Relaxation techniques are used increasingly by people in varying walks of life – not necessarily those with any form of illness. Relaxation and meditation are similar in many ways. The techniques may be different, but the ultimate goal is the same. In addition to individual therapists, who may be expensive, there are also books and tapes which provide instruction in both relaxation and meditation techniques. Many of these methods originated in the East, and have been adapted to have particular relevance for patients with cancer. Transcendental meditation was brought to the West by the Buddhists. There are a number of centres throughout Britain where you can learn the methods and spend periods in retreats with others.

Yoga is a form of exercise which pushes individuals to their own personal limits but does not involve strain and a competitive schedule. It improves fitness and teaches the ability to relax both physically and psychologically. By this means, yoga optimises the positive mental attitude and enables the individual to regain a sense of control.

The Alexander technique is a Western approach which has been the culmination of various disciplines and is widely used by people from all walks of life. There are many Alexander technique teachers and you may well find it easier to go to a class like this than to a cancer support therapist teaching similar techniques. It is similar to yoga in that it involves the development of a relaxed state of mind.

In summary, these techniques can be self-taught (although they may be better taught by a therapist) and have both physical and mental benefits. They emphasise an approach to cancer in which the mind and spirit are as important as the body in responding to the disease. You must not have unrealistic expectations of what can be achieved and any negative feelings of blame, guilt and anger which these therapies enforce are best avoided. As with any form of treatment for cancer, be it complementary or conventional, you must be the ultimate arbiter.

VISUALISATION AND HEALING

There are two broad ways in which visualisation can be used positively by cancer patients. In constructive visualisation, the disease and its individual components are imagined as other forms such as animals or inanimate objects. The patient's tumour may be given a name and the therapy which he or she is having may be imagined in an analogous form. The choice is left very much up to the individual, although the counsellor may help. One patient receiving monoclonal antibody therapy for ovarian cancer imagined the antibodies, which were labelled with radioactive isotope, as a missile which was helping her body's own resources. She imagined her body's white blood cells as goldfish which were hoovering up around her body. She saw the goldfish dressed in smart butler's uniform pushing hoovers around inside her abdomen to suck up the cancer cells. This particular patient called her disease Fred. She treated him as a friend whom she had to keep at bay, and although she did not allow herself to become angry with Fred, she knew when enough was enough!

The other form of visualisation is one used by the Chinese. In this exercise, described as bone breathing visualisation, they see the centre of the bones as responsible for the well-being of the entire body. Once in a comfortable relaxed position, they are encouraged to imagine their breath entering the body and being taken up by each of the bones in turn as the breath circulates around the body. They concentrate on the legs initially, then the legs and hands followed by the spine and ultimately the skull. The exercise is repeated, breathing in gently and then breathing out through all the bones. In this approach, visualisation is used as a means to relaxation.

Healing, like meditation, comes in many forms. Christian Science was founded at the end of the nineteenth century by Mary Baker Eddy and is based on the theory that physical illness can be overcome with faith and prayer. Spiritualism also had its origins in the nineteenth century with the establishment of a number of groups around the country. It has the happy distinction of believing that healing is favourable to atheists as well as believers. The laying on of hands, which involves the healer passing his or her hands up and down the body, is a service which is offered as a therapy by various religious organisations. It has been known to ease out pain. Descriptions of hand healing go back as far as the seventeenth century. Such a gift is thought to be possessed by very few people.

The Humanist Association works from a set of beliefs and moral ideals outside religious doctrines. Healing is available via a number of sources: a healer may be visited in his own centre, he may be contacted by post and may even visit individuals in their own homes when they are seriously ill. Whatever the means, the type of healing or the individual who administers it, it is essentially an adjunct to conventional therapy which should not be promising cures, but offering a means of maximising the individual's chances.

The Simonton technique was devised by Stephanie Simonton who has published a book entitled *The Healing Family*. It is based around a family game plan in which images of normal, everyday life can be visualised through meditation and relaxation in order to promote healing and recovery. A further book, entitled *Getting Well Again*, was written by Ms Simonton and her husband and is aimed at people with cancer. It may be useful reading for many patients who find the method of visualising images a fruitful one.

ACUPUNCTURE

This particular form of therapy originated some six thousand years ago in China. Acupuncture has been widely used for some time in the treatment of pain, including that caused by cancer, and is now offered by an increasing number of GPs who have had some training in this skill and use it in addition to conventional means. The formal training of an acupuncturist takes four years of full-time education. On your first visit the acupuncturist will want to obtain a full picture of your lifestyle, psychological stresses and diet. He will examine you thoroughly and then establish the various meridians. These are the lines through which the acupuncturist can diagnose defects in the body's systems. The approach of different individuals will vary widely, as will the degree of success. There are over a thousand medically and non-medically qualified acupuncturists in this country.

Reflexology is similar to acupuncture and deals with the release of unbalanced energies. Where an acupuncturist uses needles, a reflexologist applies gentle pressure at appropriate points to free the energy. Reflexology is conducive to relaxation and may improve your breathing.

HOMEOPATHY

Homeopathy is the science of treating a condition by the administration, usually in miniscule doses, of drugs which produce symptoms in a healthy person similar to the disease being treated. This system was founded by Samuel Hahnemann of Leipzig at the end of the eighteenth century. The assumption that 'like cures like' is contrary to any of the foundations of orthodox medicine. Homeopathy has been popular with the royal family throughout this century and there are numerous stories which support it. Prince Charles made a famous speech to the British Medical Association in

1983 in which he encouraged doctors to be more broad-minded about alternative (complementary) medicine. Small amounts of various drugs are given in a very dilute form. Consequently, it is without side effects. There are a number of NHS homeopathic centres throughout the country and many are staffed by medically qualified homeopathic physicians. Non-medically qualified practitioners are also available and can be contacted through the Society of Homeopaths.

Two points must be kept in mind:

- No homeopathist should guarantee a cure unreservedly.
- No homeopathist should demand that conventional treatment is abandoned.

Most sympathetic homeopathists will be happy to treat patients with homeopathic medicine alongside their conventional therapy. In this way homeopathy can provide a useful supportive measure for patients who find that their symptoms are not relieved by conventional treatment, even though they believe it may be the best option for their cancer.

ANTHROPOSOPHY

Anthroposophy was founded by the Austrian scientist, Rudolf Steiner, at the turn of the century. The people who practise it are all medically qualified and have additional training from the School of Spiritual Science in Switzerland. Anthroposophy is largely based around mistletoe and its special characteristics. The plant is harvested and prepared in a complicated fashion whereby male and female plants are mixed in a gravity-free centrifuge so that the extract remains biologically stable. It is then put to various uses on the host tree: mistletoe on an apple tree is believed to help the reproductive organs and breasts, whilst on an oak tree it helps the prostate. It is thought to stimulate the production of white cells and antibodies and raise the body temperature, thereby stimulating the body's defence mechanisms and protecting against cancer, making removal or treatment that much easier. Again, it must be stressed that this is not an alternative to conventional therapy for cancer. It would be very sad to forgo the beneficial effects of modern therapy in favour of a treatment which has purely anecdotal evidence to support its use.

Much of modern pharmacology is based on the use of herbs. The vinca-alkaloids are an important part of the treatment of many cancers and their source is the Madagascan periwinkle. Adriamycin was first extracted from a fungus found near to the Adriatic Sea. Herbalism is both an art and a science and forms part of the holistic approach to cancer. The herbalist uses particular groups of herbs. Some may detoxify by working on the liver, others purify the lymphatic system and there are herbs which are claimed to block the growth of cancer cells. A good herbalist working alongside a doctor may be able to help patients adapt to their situation.

One sub-group of herbalism is the Bach flower remedies. Dr Edward Bach worked in the early part of this century on preparing thirty-eight remedies from wild flowers. He was a pathologist and bacteriologist who switched to homeopathy at the turn of the century. He believed that the negative emotions in cancer patients needed to be treated and, by holding his hand over a plant, he was able to experience the properties of that plant and thereby use it to treat the individual's emotions appropriately. The therapy is completely safe and with no side effects.

DIET

The key to any diet is to adopt a sensible, balanced, healthy approach. This cannot be said of many of the diets currently recommended. Diet is a form of control whereby the patient is no longer passive in relation to his disease. The Bristol diet, which was followed more religiously when the Centre was initially established, involves three months' intensive, strict vegan diet in which 90 per cent of food must be raw in order to cleanse the body of cancer. Subsequently, the diet is relaxed, with a lesser degree of deprivation and at this point it is intended to maintain the patient's remission.

There is also a Bristol diet which is recommended in order to prevent cancer. The obvious problem with anything purporting such results is that since one in three of us are likely to develop this disease, it is not unlikely that one in three individuals adhering to the diet will feel that they have somehow failed in spite of making a Herculean effort. There are a number of aspects of the Bristol diet, and many like it recommended at different centres throughout the world, which are worrying to the orthodox physician. The word 'poisons' is frequently used for substances which many people take unavoidably throughout the course of their normal lives such as fluoride. Poison is a dangerous, emotive word which, for many people with cancer, conjures up guilt and blame, both of which are negative and destructive emotions at a time when the individual has quite enough to contend with. Vitamin supplements are also encouraged alongside the diet. If the diet is sensible and well balanced a vitamin supplement – the man-made equivalent of something which occurs naturally – should not be necessary for a normal healthy life. Eating 90 per cent raw food for three months, apart from being a severe deprivation for many people, is quite likely to be impractical. A housebound elderly person may well find it difficult to prepare his own food and cannot expect Meals-on-Wheels to serve up such diets on a regular basis! It seems logical that a person facing his biggest battle yet should feel positive and hopeful. Many of the diets recommended will make the individual feel deprived and very often they will suffer gastrointestinal symptoms which outweigh those caused by their disease.

Many alternative treatments acknowledge that diet is an essential part of the treatment of cancer and some of the more extreme suggest that the major part of the person's lifestyle that has to change. Dr Max Gerson founded the Gerson Clinic at La Gloria Hospital in Tijuana, Mexico. His theory purports that cancer is a generalised chronic degenerative disease which is a symptom of a chronically damaged body. The Gerson therapy is based on a detoxification process whereby the body is treated with minerals and organic foods, having been purged by a strict vegan diet, coffee enemas and large quantities of fresh fruit juice. This is an expensive, monotonous, intensive and time-consuming process. An individual who has been through the mill in this way may well feel that they have not only taken full control of their body, but have made a very active gesture in attempting to alter the course of their disease. But the evidence that such treatments effectively control tumour growth is slim. However, drastically changing your lifestyle may well be an effective means of coping with the psychological effects of the disease, even if it does not deal with the biological process of your cancer.

So what should you really do about diet if you have cancer? The main thing is to eat healthy balanced meals of foods you enjoy. Make sure there's plenty of roughage in the form of fibre as in brown bread and bran-containing cereals. This will avoid intestinal problems. Eat plenty of fresh fruit and lightly cooked vegetables. This should provide all the vitamins you need without resorting to artificial medication. Proponents of large doses of vitamins conveniently forget that the body just passes the excess out in the urine fairly smartly. Reduce your fat intake: avoid chips and other fried food. Experiment with different diets – you might well like vegetarian food which is delicious and easy to digest. But above all, eat what you like and feel comfortable with, rather than adhering to some rigid schedule based on any scientific sounding mumbo-jumbo.

What to eat

- Eat what you like when you want to.
- If you've lost weight, eat small meals frequently, rather than getting stuck into a single large meal every day.
- Soups are often delicious and easy to take.
- Eat plenty of fibre – brown bread, bran cereals.
- Eat lots of fresh fruit.
- Do not overcook vegetables – they will taste better and the vitamins will not be destroyed.
- Avoid too much fat – have boiled or baked potato instead of chips.
- Reduce your red meat intake – it's more difficult to digest.
- By all means stimulate the appetite with a glass of sherry or other appetiser. (Unknown to many, sherry, beer and brandy can be prescribed for this purpose in all NHS hospitals.)

CONCLUSION

If becoming completely absorbed by complementary therapy makes you feel that life is worthwhile, then why not? However, you should think of it not as an alternative to conventional medicine but as an optional extra. You must weigh up the odds yourself. If complementary therapy causes physical symptoms and makes you feel depressed and isolated, then avoid it. If you are receiving highly intensive orthodox treatment and experiencing unpleasant side effects, then complementary treatment of some sort may give you much-needed encouragement.

The saying, 'Where there's life there's hope' is never more true than for cancer sufferers. Much of the unpleasant intensive treatment involved in pursuing a cure, or a further remission from cancer, is only possible because the individual still has hope. If using complementary therapy makes you feel more hopeful, then it may be of great benefit. Some of the successes of complementary therapy appear to be almost miracle cures, which cannot be explained on any logical, scientific basis. For many people such stories provide a ray of light at the end of the tunnel and for this reason, if no other, orthodox practitioners should encourage complementary therapy alongside conventional medicine.

There are a wide range of similar forms of complementary therapy which have been devised by various individuals from both conventional and self-taught backgrounds. They provide enough fodder for an entire book in themselves, and if you are interested there is an infinite supply of reading material.

CASE HISTORY

Ruby is a middle-aged woman with two teenage children. After a six-month history of diarrhoea and some rectal bleeding, she underwent an operation and was found to have an advanced carcinoma of the colon with widespread liver and peritoneal metastases. She remained very well with a good appetite and had no weight loss. She was keen to have the best treatment available and prolong her life if at all possible. She was admitted to hospital and commenced on continuous 5-fluorouracil chemotherapy. This is a form of chemotherapy, administered as an outpatient by the patient herself. It is usually well tolerated, with very little in the way of side effects. It necessitates carrying a pump around with a syringe attached on the three days a week that the chemotherapy is given.

Ruby tolerated her chemotherapy very well initially, but then became conscious of her pump and inhibited by its continual presence as a reminder of her illness. She attended the Bristol Centre for three separate days, a month apart, and was given a vegan diet to follow. She tolerated the diet well, although she was not encouraged enthusiastically by her family, and remained well with a good appetite and no symptoms of note. She also remained on the chemotherapy. Although her blood tests implied that her liver metastases were progressing, her positive mental attitude meant that life carried on much the same for her without any outward signs of progression of her disease. Her blood tests have continued to deteriorate over the last six months, but during this time she has remained well enough to go skiing with her husband. She has returned to the Bristol Centre on a number of occasions, finding great support in sharing her experience with other cancer sufferers and in acknowledging the spiritual aspect of the human condition and the role that this has to play in dealing with cancer.

AFTER TREATMENT

It may be hard to imagine that life goes on after cancer. Many people undergo treatment while they are still experiencing the initial shock of diagnosis. When this is over, their attempt to return to a normal life is often an uphill struggle. For most patients and their families the experience of cancer, whatever its outcome, will change their lives for ever. They may have a realignment of values, their whole perspective will be changed and life itself often takes on a much more intense focus. It is important in this process that patient and family do not become victims. Initially it may be hard to view anything with a long-term perspective, but restoration to a full emotional life is every bit as important as successful therapy. If the price of cure is isolation and fear, nobody will benefit.

Having completed your course of therapy, you may attend the first follow-up clinic expecting to be told that you have been cured. Unfortunately, cancer is not like that. By the time it has been discovered, there are usually over a billion cancer cells in the body. The vast majority of these cells will have disappeared during treatment, but present-day screening techniques mean that we cannot detect even as few as 10 000 cells accurately. As a result, any doctor who tells a patient as little as one month after treatment that they have been cured is being inappropriately optimistic. It may be very likely that they have been cured, but a definite statement is not possible at this stage.

FOLLOW-UP

Follow-up clinics are useful for both you and your doctor. It may take some time to cease dreading these occasions, but as the gaps between clinics increase, reassurance comes. The clinic is there as a safety net to which you can return if your symptoms recur, or fears about the disease become overwhelming. The most important fact your doctor can learn from a follow-up clinic is how you are feeling. Blood tests, X-rays and other investigations may be an important part of monitoring but a very well patient with no symptoms is unlikely to have a recurrence. On the other hand, someone who is depressed, has become obsessed with their disease and is completely unable to return to a normal life, needs encouragement and reassurance.

The follow-up visit usually begins with a discussion about any symptoms. The doctor will then examine you and arrange for any necessary tests to be carried out. In cancers where any recurrence or spread of the disease is likely to respond well to treatment, tests will be done to ensure that any problems can be detected at an early stage. In such malignancies blood tests, X-rays and scans are important and they will be a regular part of the patient's review. With other cancers tests will not be carried out unless there are obvious worrying symptoms. You should not feel that you are being neglected simply because an investigation is not performed. Ideally most patients would hope to reach a point where visits are necessary only once or twice a year.

GETTING BACK TO WORK

The diagnosis of cancer is likely to be followed by an operation, or at least a biopsy, then radiotherapy and/or chemotherapy. It may well be three or four months before you feel well enough to return to work, although some people manage to work throughout their radiotherapy or chemotherapy, only missing the part of the day taken up by treatment, or short admissions to receive drugs.

Your GP can advise and provide the necessary certificates. Statutory sick pay is provided by your employer for up to twenty-eight weeks of illness. After this time, you switch to invalidity benefit paid by the State. The hospital social worker will be familiar with all the ins and outs of sorting out sick pay and should be contacted if problems arise.

Once employers are aware of the reasons for your absence, they may have their own ideas about your subsequent ability to do your job. It is essential to enlist the support and help of your medical staff and GP at this point. Any specific disability can be anticipated. If certain tasks associated with your job are impossible, it may be feasible to amend your job so that you can cope. However, there is no reason why most people cannot resume full employment exactly as before once they have had a chance to regain their strength. Getting back to work is the most important factor in returning to a normal life and much of your self-esteem is likely to depend on this.

If you have any specific difficulties in relation to your job or employer, you should air these in the clinic. An explanatory letter from the doctor concerned will often do much to dispel any fears and misconceptions. It is not only patients with cancer who fear the disease: its taboos extend to people close to that person. Irrational behaviour from family, friends and work colleagues is not unusual and the only way this can be countered is to avoid mystery and replace it with understanding.

FINANCIAL PROBLEMS

These can be divided into short and longer term problems. The latter include returning to full-time employment, the possibility of ultimate invalidity and the fear of having a surviving family inadequately cared for. All of us, whether in full health, young or old, with or without dependants, should make a will. If this has not been done before the diagnosis of cancer, it should be as soon as possible thereafter. However uncomplicated the will, it is probably best to consult a solicitor when drawing it up so as to avoid misunderstandings between the beneficiaries. For most patients, unless the will is complex, the expense of a solicitor will not be very great.

Not only will everyone be assured of the legalities, but a solicitor's advice on ways to minimise estate duties could save a lot of money.

As far as the short term is concerned the financial support you receive during your treatment will vary from employer to employer. Most people are entitled to government-funded sick pay and, if the period of illness continues, possibly sickness benefit or invalidity benefit as well. This is likely to fall short of your usual income and most people will be keen to return to work as soon as possible.

Social services can often help with unexpected expenses, which may arise shortly after a diagnosis has been made. Many people find the idea of having a social worker allocated to them is somehow rather shameful, as if they are 'problem' cases who can't cope, and will not ask for these services until they are desperate. This is unfortunate since social workers can often help out at an early stage and avoid any later crises. They are also able to advise about contributions from special funds for cancer patients and which sources to approach for expenses such as fares and accommodation, and for obtaining free prescriptions and attendance allowances where appropriate. The Cancer Relief MacMillan Fund has an annual budget of £1.5 million which is distributed to patients in need, particularly for help in getting to hospital for treatment and follow-up appointments, and for families to visit patients. For children with cancer, the Malcolm Sargent Fund serves the same purpose.

If you need to be cared for at home at any point, your family may be entitled to an attendance allowance or a care allowance. You can get details of who to claim from, and when and how to claim, most easily through the social worker. Patients with a colostomy, ileostomy or urostomy are all entitled to free prescriptions – not only for anything to do with their operation but for any other drugs or dressings they may need. For men under 65 and women under 60 who are in full-time employment and not entitled to free prescriptions, it may be best to purchase a 'season ticket', for approximately £12, which will cover all their prescriptions for three months. It is worth asking your doctor whether this is likely to be an advantage or whether a long-term repeat prescription might be cheaper.

In the long term, you may find you are no longer able to pay your mortgage or insurance. If you can't go back to work, your mortgage payments will be subject to the same restrictions as anybody on statutory sick pay or sickness benefit. As for life insurance, the people who do not have to worry are those who are already adequately covered. If you are thinking about taking out a new life insurance policy after treatment, it is worth contacting the Association of British Insurers (see chapter 10) to ask for a list of insurers who look favourably on people who have recently had a diagnosis of cancer. It may then be possible to shop around to compare their rates, or alternatively wait for a period of one year, when rates may be more favourable still. Often insurers will reduce their rates as the disease-free interval increases and it is worth keeping this in mind and enquiring regularly. Once again, information from your doctor as to the nature of your diagnosis, stage of disease and your likely prognosis will be essential to obtain insurance. The content of the letter should be discussed with you, both from the point of view of understanding your likely prognosis and whether the doctor feels you are a reasonable risk for life assurance.

Drawing-up and making funeral arrangements is probably best discussed when it is least likely to be particularly relevant. The social worker may be a useful means of support and, if special funds are needed, these can be obtained at the relevant time from a number of the cancer charities. Alternatively, you may prefer to set a sum of money aside to take the burden away from your family. The subject of cremation or burial is probably difficult to approach but it may be a source of comfort for the relatives, should the occasion arise, that the ceremony is according to the wishes of their loved one.

TALKING TO OTHERS

This is something that will happen from an early stage in your treatment. You will meet other patients in the chemotherapy clinic, whilst waiting for radiotherapy treatment and on the ward after surgery. They will be at varying stages with their disease and will have very different stories of their experiences. This can sometimes be confusing and it may help to approach a specific support group. This could be a general one such as BACUP (British Association of Cancer United Patients) or CancerLink, or alternatively, a charity used to dealing with one particular type of cancer. Many of the bigger charities and organisations have a help line which is manned at least part of the week and may have regular local association meetings. They may publish pamphlets about particular illnesses which can provide information in greater clarity and detail than it is possible to glean from the doctor at the clinic. In addition, you can get support from the hospital treating you, with care continuing after your discharge from hospital and after the completion of your treatment. This supplements home visits from the district nurse, GP nurse or other paramedical staff.

Many people who have recently been diagnosed as having cancer will feel angry and very frightened. By meeting others in a similar position, especially those who are further down the road with their disease, you can see how they cope. We are all different, however, and you must keep this in mind when comparing your own experiences to those of others. You should not feel a failure if your illness does not progress as well as someone else's. At times, the information you obtain from different sources can be conflicting and it is then important to ask your specialist to act as arbiter. If you are not happy about your management and feel that you have not explored all the possible avenues, then ask for a second opinion. This is, and always has been, readily available under the NHS. Don't believe that you have to pay for private treatment in order to be sure of obtaining the best.

RECURRENT DISEASE

The ultimate fear of most patients is that their cancer will return. As time goes by so the risk of recurrence decreases and your follow-up visits to the clinic will therefore become less frequent. Of course, the chances of recurrence depend on what type of cancer you have had and how far it had spread when you were first treated. Some highly aggressive cancers will probably recur within two years of diagnosis if they are going to recur at all and, if you have been disease-free for five years, the likelihood is that you have in fact been cured. On the other hand, there are diseases which respond to primary treatment, but many years later, cells that have spread from the primary site begin to grow, causing problems again. Many cancers, possibly up to half, can still be cured at the time of diagnosis. These include those which are sensitive to hormone therapy (e.g. breast cancer and prostatic· cancer), those which can be cured by chemotherapy (e.g. lymphomas and testicular tumours) or those where the only problem is a local recurrence and further surgery or radiotherapy is able to control this disease without it spreading further.

Although some cancers cannot be cured, this may not in fact reduce the patient's life expectancy. Many patients live with their cancer for many years. It causes little in the way of symptoms and they are quite often able to reach a normal life expectancy. Other patients may have numerus recurrences of their malignancy, with the periods of remission between recurrences being of a reasonable length.

It is also important to maintain a balance between the length of time the patient is expected to survive and their quality of life. If someone is expected to live only a few months, even with treatment, and the treatment itself is likely to cause unpleasant side effects, then the patient's quality of life – and personal dignity – would obviously suffer. For this reason, any decision about further treatment should take into consideration possible side effects, the chances of good periods of remission, the number of clinic visits involved and the likely outcome. Since the implications for the patient are far greater than for the doctor, the doctor must be aware of the patient's priorities.

One common misconception about further treatment is that it is unlimited. If radical radiotherapy has already been given, the normal tissue in that area will probably not be able to withstand any further dose without being irreparably damaged. Most tumours are sensitive to only a limited number of drugs, and once these have been exhausted, options become increasingly limited. Furthermore, both radiotherapy and chemotherapy are toxic to the bone marrow stem cells and in patients who have already received intensive treatment, further treatment may result in prolonged bone marrow suppression. This means that the reproduction of white blood cells (which fight infection) and platelets (one of the factors involved in blood clotting) will be lowered, leaving the patient at greater risk of infection, spontaneous bruising and bleeding. As a result, patients may require frequent stays in hospital for antibiotics to treat or prevent infections, or platelet transfusions if these are low. Bone marrow suppression is the most common problem that limits further treatment, but damage to the kidneys, the nerves (both those in the spinal cord and those supplying the limbs), the small intestine and the lungs can all result from chemotherapy or radiotherapy to certain parts of the body. Further treatment can cause as many problems to the patient as the recurrence of the disease.

PAIN CONTROL

One of the great fears of any cancer patient is pain. Part of the taboo stems from a fear that their last few months will be spent in uncontrolled pain. In fact virtually half of the patients who die with cancer never experience pain at any point. Moreover, with increased understanding of cancer, we can now anticipate the problem. By making frequent adjustments the correct balance can be attained to give good pain control twenty-four hours a day without causing undue sleepiness. It may be difficult to cure all cancers, but there can be no excuses for allowing people to suffer pain. Analgesics (pain-killers) are given regularly so that pain never breaks through to the surface. Usually, patients will be given a pain killer such as paracetamol to start with and, if this is not enough, moved onto a combination analgesic which contains paracetamol and another more powerful drug.

Anti-inflammatory tablets such as aspirin can also be used – these can be particularly helpful with bone pain. If they fail to control pain adequately, the opiate family of drugs are used. These are drugs derived from opium – an extract of the poppy. Dihydrocodeine or codeine are likely to be the first opiates used. Subsequently morphine and diamorphine are the mainstay of pain control. Sadly, morphine is often thought of as a drug which is only given to patients when they are about to die. This is far from the truth. Indeed, some drugs such as slow-release morphine preparations (like MST) can be used by patients with severe pain for many years. As for opiates being addictive, there is little to support this theory unless they are injected directly into a vein. In fact, if the patient is experiencing pain they are badly needed and can be reduced fairly rapidly once the pain has resolved. It is only when patients have been on opiate drugs for more than a period of weeks that they cannot be withdrawn suddenly.

The fear of using opiate analgesics is not unique to patients, and there are some doctors who are reluctant to use such treatment. In fact, opiates are remarkably safe. Many of the problems experienced by drug abusers using opiates are the result of infections from unhygienic needles and syringes. For pain control, these drugs are usually given in tablet or syrup form and are much less addictive.

Morphine is said to shorten patients' lives, but there are no observations to support this idea. Someone who is in severe pain and persistently distressed is more likely to have a rapid, unhappy demise than a patient with good pain control who is able to lead a peaceful and calm life in his own surroundings. Opiates only cause hallucinations if they are given in large doses and they should not be withheld on the grounds that the patient is not sufficiently unwell or in pain, to justify them. As long as they are started at a relatively low dose, they can be matched to the level of pain. Some individuals are particularly sensitive to opiates and by starting at a low dose, this can be detected. If undue drowsiness results, the tablets are simply stopped.

How pain-killers are given

In patients who require frequent doses of analgesics which vary widely from day to day, it may be best to change to using a small pump. A tiny needle is inserted just under the skin and supplies a continuous infusion of the drug from a syringe fixed in a small, battery-operated or clockwork pump. There is no real difference between morphine and diamorphine, apart from the actual dose required, although the latter is more soluble and is more likely to be used when given as an infusion. This is ideal for patients who are nursed at home, since the patient or member of the family can be taught to site the fine needle under the skin themselves and make up the drug so that the syringe can be changed once a day. This form of pain control has really helped to make life much more tolerable.

Occasionally patients have such severe pain that the doses of opiates required are sufficient to impair their level of consciousness. In this situation, the drug can be administered directly into the fluid surrounding the spinal cord. A catheter is inserted by an anaesthetist in much the same way as an epidural catheter is used for women in labour. The cannula in the spine is held in place and a small reservoir is attached outside. When the patient has particularly severe pain and needs an extra dose of the drug, he can press the reservoir and a top-up dose will be delivered. This relatively new form of pain control has not been used widely outside hospital as yet.

In addition to drugs, treatment itself can constitute a form of pain control. For boney pain and some painful skin lesions a single dose of radiotherapy can alleviate the symptoms for a considerable time. Patients with widespread bony metastases may be admitted to hospital overnight and given a single dose of radiotherapy to the lower or upper half of the body. With sedation and drugs to control sickness, the patient usually sleeps through the experience and any of the other side effects. For more

---

CONTROLLING PAIN

- Simple painkillers – aspirin, paracetamol.
- More potent analgesics – codyramol, coproxamol, cocodamol, dihydrocodeine, distalgesic.
- Anti-inflammatory drugs – indomethacin, naproxen.
- Synthetic morphine-like drugs – palfium, diconal, fortral.
- Morphine and diamorphine given by mouth or by injection.
- Many drugs are made by several manufacturers and have different trade names which adds to confusion – your doctor can advise.
- Whichever drugs are used, remember you get no medals for being able to withstand pain.
- Your doctor (GP or hospital) can advise about how best to time pain control medicine.

localised secondaries, a short course of radiotherapy will often shrink the lesion causing the pain, and patients may find that their regular analgesics can be tailed off. Similarly, chemotherapy, while not used for pain control, will automatically lessen pain if it reduces a painful site of the disease.

DYING AND BEREAVEMENT

Once death has been accepted as inevitable, there has to be a change of approach by the doctors and nurses in relation to care and communication. This transition is often difficult to make within the hospital environment, since the staff have to look after potentially curable patients simultaneously. Consequently, there is a tendency for dying patients to be placed in a side-ward, and visited by the staff when necessary, but not spontaneously. Sixty per cent of the population in Great Britain die in hospital, and even more in the United States. Sadly this figure has increased in the last two decades.

The hospice movement

The first form of care for the dying, which we now take for granted, was seen in the Middle Ages. At that time hospices were run by religious organisations. In the nineteenth century Mary Aikenhead opened the first modern hospice in Dublin. She founded the Irish Sisters of Charity and one of their tasks was to care for the dying. From her experiences, she decided that a nursing home was needed for dying patients that was quieter and smaller than a hospital for the acutely ill. She used her own house initially and adopted the name of the resting places to the Holy Land, 'Hospice'. At the beginning of the twentieth century the Sisters opened St Joseph's Hospice in Hackney, London. Subsequently, two further hospices were founded in London and in 1899 an order of Dominican nuns had founded the first hospice in New York City.

Since that time there has been a great expansion in continuing care, and Britain now leads the world in terms of provision both for people dying in hospices and for those who wish to die at home. Although most of the early hospices were founded by religious orders, many NHS hospices have no particular denominational leaning.

There are a number of advantages to hospice care. Many of these are for the relatives who may be exhausted or anxious or attempting to hold down full-time employment. Many dying patients live alone and are too weak to cope. They may require specific medication or treatment that cannot be easily given at home. Many cancer patients are old and may not have relatives nearby. In addition, brave families who are doing their best to cope may benefit from short periods of respite care to allow them to recuperate. If there are particular complications of the patient's illness which are better cared for in the hospice and the family would like to be near the dying patient, it is usually possible to arrange for relatives to stay.

Dying at home

A high proportion of more than 40 000 people who die at home in Britain do not need any particular support. However, there is a significant minority who, without the support of a continuing care team, would need admission to an institution. After a survey instigated by the Marie Curie Foundation in the early 1950s, the needs of cancer patients and their relatives for adequate support was highlighted. In 1958 a 'day-and-night nursing service' was introduced. Sadly the availability of such services varies widely from region to region and, with the current financial constraints on the NHS, many have been reduced. In 1973 a nurse and doctor from St Joseph's Hospice began to visit dying patients at home. At that time, the GPs were responsible for home support, with the aid of district nurses. In 1975 St Joseph's Hospice established a service called MacMillan Nurses which in its first three years cared for 1000 patients dying from cancer. Many of these were able to spend most of their remaining weeks at home. This has led to the current situation where more than 60 per cent of St Joseph's dying patients are at home. The lynch-pins of this type of home care team are the nurses. The number of visits they make will vary but, where necessary, patients are visited up to eight times daily. In addition there are doctors, social workers and physiotherapists available, all of whom contribute to keeping the patients at home for as long as is possible.

Such continuing care at home will vary geographically and is likely to be better where there is a hospice nearby. The hospital specialist, GP and social worker should all be able to inform the patient and family about the services available and a determined family who feel strongly that the patient should be able to die at home should express this wish as early as possible. The advantages of dying at home are evident. The patient is in familiar surroundings, he has a chance to spend time with his relatives and is able to maintain both dignity and individuality. He is not lost in the anonymity of dying as a hospital or hospice inpatient and the bereavement process is likely to be kinder.

If the final stage of the patient's illness is relatively long, it is worth exploring the possibility of installing gadgets and appliances to improve the quality of life and leave the family more independent. Cancer is an emotive disease which attracts more money for charity than any other. Consequently, a well-informed social worker will be able to direct the family to a number of different sources for grants to help with appliances, fares and numerous other items of expenditure which might not otherwise be manageable.

BEREAVEMENT

Whenever someone dies from whatever cause their friends and relatives go through the process of bereavement. How long it will last and how severe the grief will depend on the closeness to the person who has died and their ability to cope with their own reactions. Time is a great healer in this respect. Many events resulting in disappointment are difficult to take at first. Even failing your driving test, not getting a job after an interview, or failing an exam at school may fill you with despondency and gloom. A few years later these events are forgotten. In the same way the process of bereavement allows you to adapt to the fact that a loved one will no longer be there and that life will have to change to meet the new circumstances. However long the terminal phase of the illness there will be a reaction of grief, although a long illness may provide an opportunity for many of the

stages of bereavement to be experienced by patient and family simultaneously. The one stage which almost invariably does not occur before
death is acceptance.

The commonest emotion experienced by all of us will be grief. This may
be preceded by short periods of shock and numbness when it is difficult to
accept or fully absorb the implications. Subsequently, we are likely to feel
desperate and sad, with a feeling of futility about life. We may retreat into
ourselves with apathy, which is expressed in both mental and physical
symptoms, withdrawing generally from society. Some people may be very
agitated and restless, with no appetite and unable to sleep, and this may
itself be coupled with feelings of self-doubt and guilt about the death of
the loved one. They may find elaborate ways of blaming themselves for
what has happened, or feel guilty about the way they behaved towards the
dying person. Along with feelings of self-reproach, they may feel that
others involved in caring for their loved one during the final illness are to
blame.

Although we are all very different in our reactions, some components of
grief are fairly predictable. It often helps to understand that we are not
alone in our feelings. One problem that arises time and time again is the
wish to have had a better relationship with the person who has died. If only
we had done those things they wanted to do, gone on that holiday, bought
that caravan, been less critical of their quirks. These feelings may take some
months to disappear.

Sometimes we may deny that death has actually occurred. We may talk
about things as though they were alive and even make plans as though
nothing has happened. Until death is accepted it is difficult to reconcile
the situation so that normal life can be resumed.

Severe grief reactions are usually considered as those which are particularly long. There is no accepted 'normal' period of mourning. Somewhere
between six and twelve months is the usual time, the period being longer
where the relationship was longer. Periods of grief may be suppressed for
some time, only to return on specific occasions such as a birthday, anniversary or the anniversary of the death itself. People who have experienced
frequent losses may develop blunted responses. This was seen during the

last two world wars. This blunting also occurs in children who have lost a parent. They are able to subdue their grief and, as a result, deny a need for affection. This may interfere with their emotional development and can sometimes cause problems in later life.

Those who lose people with cancer may experience an extreme fear of the disease – a reaction which may be even more likely if attempts have been made to avoid mentioning the disease and its effects. The development of symptoms similar to those suffered by the patient may also be a form of mourning. Consciously or unconsciously the mourner may be taking on their characterisation in an attempt to keep their memory alive.

Severe bereavement reactions are not predictable. They appear to be more common in women, particularly those who are young or middle-aged when widowed, or those who have lost children. Whatever the mechanisms, their complexities and the period of mourning, it is an inevitable part of the loss associated with bereavement. It is a natural process and only if it impairs an ability to return to normal life after a period should it be considered as abnormal. Whatever the reaction, it may be helped by professional support or perhaps a support group with people who have endured a similar experience. Having worked through the emotions provoked by the bereavement, the mature adult can accept these emotions

Hints to overcome the loss of a close friend or relative with cancer

- Don't hold back the tears – let emotion flow.
- Don't be afraid to talk about their illness to others.
- If you have specific worries about their final illness, ask the doctors to tell you what happened.
- Think about the good times as well as their last stages of life.
- Try to get back to a normal routine as soon as possible – back to work, sorting out the house and so on.
- Develop new interests – they wouldn't want you to sit around and mope.
- If you have a faith, seek spiritual guidance.
- If you have trouble sleeping, tell your GP. A short course of sleeping pills could help you cope.

and find a balance where he can adjust to his new life with those left behind.

CASE HISTORIES

1 Barbara

At the age of fifty-eight, Barbara was diagnosed as having breast cancer. Two years later she developed pain in her spine and it was found that the disease had spread. She was given the drug tamoxifen (a hormonal agent) and initially both her pain and the spread of the disease improved. Nine months later the pain had returned and she was switched to an alternative hormone therapy (Provera – a progestogen). This had only a short-lived response and thereafter she was given a course of chemotherapy. Over the next two years she continued to remit and relapse, and was given short courses of mild chemotherapy when her symptoms became too severe.

Then she developed severe pains in her left hip and over a short period of time a fracture of the neck of her left femur became apparent. By this time her blood count was low as a result of extensive radiotherapy and chemotherapy and it was also suspected that the cancer was invading her bone marrow, reducing the number of white blood cells being produced. Her bone abnormalities on the X-ray were now so widespread that even if the left hip were repaired it was likely that her spine would be the next problem. Since Barbara could no longer tolerate radiotherapy to her lumbar spine, and had exhausted the range of drugs available, there was little left to be offered in the way of conventional treatment.

Her left hip was operated on, fusing the thigh bone to the pelvis so that she could be transferred from bed to chair without pain. By this time she was being nursed on a special type of bed (a Clinitron). This consists of a series of beads that float on a cushion of air in which the patient can be turned with minimal effort by the nurses, and without discomfort for the patient. Having recovered from the hip operation it was possible to organise this special type of bed at home, with the local health authority funding the hiring costs. Barbara was transferred home with maximum support from the district nurse, continuing care team, her husband and son and with a bed on the same floor as her bathroom. She was successfully nursed for some weeks until she died.

2 John

John, a seventy-eight-year-old man, came to the casualty department with a chest infection, having recently coughed up some blood. His chest X-ray was abnormal, showing enlarged lymph nodes and a mass visible in the right lung. It was felt that it was highly likely he had a carcinoma. Three attempts were made to obtain a biopsy, but all were unsuccessful. The likely diagnosis and his chances of survival were explained to John. He was eventually discharged home, but had no next of kin and was not able to cope. The continuing care team were involved and, although his physical health remained relatively stable, he became increasingly depressed. It was felt that he was likely to live for some months yet and an application was made for him to be admitted to St Joseph's Hospice. In the hospice he had the company of other people in a similar position. He was able to discuss his diagnosis and its implications and, after a year in the company of his new-found friends, John's entire approach to life had improved. He became optimistic and determined to fight the disease, and eventually gained enough confidence to discharge himself from the hospice. It is now two years since he left St Joseph's Hospice. His chest X-ray is still abnormal, but the disease has not progressed and his general health is stable with only mild chest symptoms. John may well have been cured; it is possible that he was even misdiagnosed in the first place since no definite evidence was obtained. Whatever his health, it is apparent that it has been paralleled by his state of mind. Such 'miracles' may constitute less than 1 per cent of all patients. There is no formula, rhyme or reason for this outcome but it provides a hopeful note for those patients who fear a terminal phase in their illness.

THE FUTURE

SOME TALL STORIES – BREAKTHROUGHS AND REALITY

One of the biggest problems facing doctors treating cancer is false hopes raised by so-called breakthroughs. These occur with monotonous regularity and are often first published in Sunday newspapers. There is considerable media interest in all cancer treatments, especially those which are sensational. Furthermore, cancer research is funded by charities which have to collect money in competition with an ever-growing list of good causes. Charities have become much more business-like in their approach to the collection of funds and it is not surprising that any advances in research will be maximised by their public relations department. The stories are usually put out honestly and without exaggeration; but just as messages get twisted when repeated by different people, so cancer cure stories tend to be exaggerated. False hopes are raised, and this can add greatly to the distress of relatives and friends of patients who later find out that their hopes were groundless. There is the sad sight of hundreds of patients embarked on an Odyssey, searching for the latest miracle cure. A company has even been started in the USA to cater for people wanting experimental treatments that may be difficult to obtain.

The best person to advise you about novel treatments is your oncologist. To go searching for experimental treatment without at least discussing it with him would be foolish. One of the greatest problems in investigating any new type of treatment is how to assess its effects on tumour growth. In order to see what effect a treatment is having, the tumour must be measurable. Even in patients with widespread cancer, this may not be possible and, for this reason, many patients are not suitable for experimental treatments.

IS THERE ANYTHING I CAN DO NOW?

This is a common question asked by many patients with cancer when conventional avenues have been fully explored. We have discussed the various complementary approaches, none of which offers miracle cures, but may have considerable supportive benefit. The best person to advise is your consultant. He will know what is available and how you can obtain it. Further information can be obtained from cancer information services such as BACUP or CancerLink.

If, after discussing it with your consultant, you are really concerned that you are not getting a chance to take part in a clinical study appropriate for your disease, ask to be referred for a second opinion. This service is quite free in the NHS, but surprisingly few patients avail themselves of it. One of the great attractions of the British system of health care is the GP, who can act as a filter of information and an agent for the patient, guiding and helping with treatment decisions. As cancer treatment becomes more complex, having such a counsellor is vital. It is therefore important that you have a GP whom you can trust and whose opinion you value. He is in the best position to assess on your behalf the likelihood of a new treatment being successful for you. New treatments are usually given in centres involved in teaching and research at the medical schools throughout the country. They are rarely performed in smaller centres.

How to be sure that everything possible has been done

- Discuss possible investigational treatments with your consultant.
- See your GP.
- Ask for a second opinion from another consultant (this can be either a private or NHS appointment).

- Contact BACUP or CancerLink.
- If you hear about a new treatment, write directly to the investigator.

CLINICAL TRIALS

How do doctors know that a treatment is likely to work? New drugs and types of radiation have all to be tested out on real patients. A clinical trial is the main way of assessing a new treatment and is an essential part of trying to improve the treatment offered. With some drugs the result is so striking that little more needs to be done. Penicillin for pneumonia is a good example. But for nearly all anti-cancer drugs the problem is more complex requiring detailed analysis of results in hundreds of people. Sometimes there are several ways of treating a particular type of cancer. The clearest way to sort out which is best is to split the patients into groups randomly, treat them and compare the results afterwards.

Until a decade ago such randomised trials were carried out on cancer patients, often without them knowing their own diagnosis and certainly without them being told that they were being randomly divided into two different treatment groups. The argument against informing the patient is that it might be a shock if a doctor honestly told a patient he was going to decide treatment by the flip of a coin. Patients want to respect and have confidence in their doctor's judgement. Imagine the captain of a jumbo jet announcing he was about to toss a coin to tell him which runway to land on as he was not sure which was best. I suspect you would change airlines!

Despite its problems, the randomised trial is often the only way to solve many issues about cancer treatment. In breast cancer there are many different operations that can be performed, from simply removing the lump followed by radiotherapy, down to the most cosmetically disfiguring operations. For many years it was unclear which procedure produced the best results. Surgeons and radiotherapists all over the world claimed that their own way of treating breast cancer was the best. Randomised trials have sorted out the issue: the type of surgery performed for early breast cancer makes no difference to the patient's chances of survival, and therefore should be that which is the least disturbing to her.

The questions which still require randomised trials include the role of chemotherapy in breast and other types of tumour after the cancer has been removed surgically. This type of chemotherapy is given in the hope of killing any microscopic deposits at the time the primary site is treated. However logical the use of such treatment, it does have side effects. It is important that we determine as quickly as possible which groups of patients are best suited to which drugs. Again, only randomised trials can answer such questions.

Some trials have used historical controls. This means comparing a new treatment with one used in patients treated in the past. Unfortunately, such trials may be of little value as our ability to classify a disease can change dramatically over a period of a few years. During the 1970s scientists studied the use of interferon in children with osteosarcoma – a bone tumour. Children receiving interferon for eighteen months after amputation were compared with children in the previous three years who had no interferon. A dramatic improvement was noted with interferon, and the drug was widely recommended. But we now know that there is no difference between patients treated with interferon and those treated without it. The reason for this is that before the early 1970s, chest tomography and CT scanning were not performed. This meant that in many of the children who were thought to have disease localised in the amputated limb, the disease had in fact spread elsewhere. In the later group of children, the diagnosis was much more accurate and amputation was only carried out if the disease was restricted to one area.

ETHICS

Most hospitals in Europe and in the USA have a review committee to consider the ethics of any investigation. This consists of doctors specialising in different areas, lay people, members of the religious community and a lawyer. If necessary, the investigator wishing to carry them through may be asked to justify his actions. Most of the trials considered by the ethics committee are straightforward and have clear benefits for the patients. Others may not be so clear.

A good illustration occurred in Birmingham in 1985 when a randomised study of the infusion of a drug, 5-fluorouracil, was carried out in patients with colon cancer which had spread to the liver. The study aimed to find out whether there was any benefit to be had from infusing the drug directly into the vein supplying the liver. Unfortunately, the patients were not told that they were going to be randomised. The relative of one patient who subsequently died complained. Most ethical committees now insist that the patients be informed of randomisation, and consent in writing to any study. Of course this means that a full and frank discussion is necessary between doctors and patient before any treatment can begin. This alone is a good thing.

Despite all the hullabaloo about ethics in medicine, virtually no doctor would deliberately harm a patient or put their life at risk. It comes down to a matter of trust between doctor and patient. Without such trust, cancer treatment, whether conventional or experimental, is a difficult business.

SOME NEW DIRECTIONS

Monoclonal antibodies

These are produced by immunising animals with a very small amount of tumour and collecting those antibodies that react against it. These antibodies are immortalised in special cell cultures which grow indefinitely in the laboratory. They can be used to help classify tumours, making the diagnosis more precise, and also as potential 'magic bullets' for treatment. Monoclonal antibodies have been used to discover new tumour markers for ovarian, pancreatic and lung cancer which give a good indication of how a patient is doing. If the patient is responding, then it may be possible to reduce the intensity of treatment. If they are not, it may need to be increased. In ovarian cancer, where chemotherapy can be effective but unfortunately has rather unpleasant side effects, tumour markers can help in choosing the number of cycles of treatment to be given.

Sometimes it is very difficult for doctors to tell in the laboratory which type of tumour a patient has or the exact site of a primary tumour. This knowledge is vital in choosing whether to treat it by drugs, radiotherapy or surgery. A mixture of monoclonal antibodies active against a variety of types of cancer is used on the tumour and the particular type that shows up in large quantities in the tests tells the doctor what type of primary cancer the patient has.

CASE HISTORY

A 32-year-old man went to his GP with a lump in the left side of his neck. He was sent up to the hospital outpatients department where he was seen by a surgeon who organised some blood tests and a chest X-ray, and brought him into hospital for a biopsy. The blood tests and X-ray were normal, but the biopsy caused confusion in the pathology laboratory. One pathologist thought it was a testicular tumour and the other a lymphoma. A third opinion was obtained from another hospital: the pathologist here thought it looked like lung cancer. The patient was seen by an oncologist, who was placed in something of a dilemma. Both testicular cancer and lymphoma should be curable, but the drugs needed are different for each disease. If the tumour was from the lung, on the other hand, then where was the primary? It is less likely to be treated successfully. How can he advise the patient without the information?

The tumour was sent to a reference laboratory where monoclonal antibodies were used to decide what type it was. The results showed staining consistent with an antibody raised against a testicular tumour. The patient had a tumour of his testis, even though clinical examination of his testes was completely normal. He was given chemotherapy using a three-drug combination and now, four years later, is alive and well.

Monoclonals also have other diagnostic uses. They can be injected into patients in tracer quantities linked to a small radioactive marker, usually radiolabelled iodine or indium. These two agents can be picked up on the scanners that are available in most hospitals. Thus, it is possible to obtain an image of the tumour throughout the body with one simple scan. So far, it has been difficult to show that monoclonal scanning is better than conventional X-rays. But it may be simpler, and a one-stage process, to detect cancer. The antibody is given into an arm or a leg, and then after a few hours homes in on the tumour. Any unbound antibody is excreted either through the liver or kidney and an image of the patient can then be made. Such information may be very valuable in deciding whether to perform an aggressive type of operation. If the disease has spread, then clearly such a procedure may be futile.

In the future it may be possible to use the antibodies as 'magic bullets' seeking out the tumour like guided missiles. If the antibodies are given 'warheads' of a poison such as ricin (a very potent poison derived from a bean plant), they could be used to kill tumour cells. Clinical trials are already going on using ricin-labelled antibodies but the results are not very promising yet because at the moment less than 1 per cent of the antibody given into a vein ends up in the tumour. Also, because the antibodies come from another animal, our own immune system tries to destroy them. Both these problems need to be overcome before the research can produce better results.

Antibody-guided radiotherapy using an antibody coupled to a powerful radioactive warhead, suffers the same drawbacks. There are some circumstances, however, where it may be possible to use existing antibodies. When a cancer is spreading in a body cavity, such as the peritoneum in the abdomen, or the pleural space in the chest, it may be possible to inject an antibody, labelled with a suitable isotope, directly into the space. The antibody will increase the radiation dose given to tumour cells without causing side effects. Trials of this type of irradiation are currently in progress.

Interferon and interleukin

These are two of the many communication molecules of the body's immune system. They allow the white cells that are involved in defending us from infection, and sometimes cancer, to talk to each other. Interferon is produced by cells infected with virus and will block subsequent infection by other viruses. The discovery of how to isolate interferon marked a breakthrough in anti-viral research, but the problem was that large numbers of human white cells had to be used to prepare it. The solution came in 1980 when interferon was produced by genetic engineering. This led to clinical trials in a whole range of diseases. Unfortunately, interferon has had little impact in cancer treatment. Very few diseases have been found to respond to it. Hairy cell leukaemia, the tumour type which responds best to it, is incredibly rare, with only about 100 cases per year occurring in the whole of the UK. Interferon may have a role in the treatment of chronic myeloid leukaemia, certain types of lymphoma and some AIDS-related cancers; but how it works is still a great mystery.

There has been considerable excitement recently about the discovery that some interleukins produce dramatic responses in cancer patients. Interleukins are released by cells of the immune system. The most intensively investigated is interleukin 2 (IL-2), which stimulates T-lymphocytes – the sort that kill other cells. IL-2 has now been given to many patients with different tumours and responses have been seen: mainly in kidney cancer and melanoma, two diseases notoriously difficult to treat with chemotherapy.

The cells involved in destroying tumour cells are called lymphokine activated killer (LAK) cells. LAK cells may not be the only way in which IL-2 works. Lymphocytes can often be found infiltrating a tumour. These can be collected at the time of surgery and stimulated by IL-2. After several days the cells can be given back to the patient. Rather surprisingly, they always seem to home in on an area of tumour. These lymphocytes, stimulated by IL-2, can produce further responses, even in patients who do not respond to IL-2 alone. Clearly, we seem to be on the threshold of some exciting new advances.

Oncogenes

One of the most exciting recent discoveries has been that of cancer-related genes – oncogenes. Cancer is the enemy within – the cell, with all its intricate control processes, goes wrong and causes chaos. For many years viruses – the smallest type of living organism – had been known to cause certain cancers in some animals such as mice, cats, rats and chimpanzees.

But there was no evidence that these viruses were very relevant to us. Nevertheless, scientists began studying how these viruses caused cancer in animals and in cells growing in the laboratory.

The experiment was simple: a single layer of cells growing in tissue culture was infected with virus. The cells suddenly started to undergo cell division and pile up on each other. Normal cells stop growing when they touch each other in tissue culture but cancer cells do not. Scientists then began analysing the molecules which caused cells to become malignant. They made changes to the structure of the virus and found there was a single gene responsible for malignant transformation. This was called the **oncogene**.

There are now some fifty known oncogenes. Interest in these fascinating pieces of genetic information grew with the advent of gene cloning in the late 1970s. Many of the genes were cloned and a very surprising observation was made: perfectly normal animal and human DNA, the genetic material we all possess, contains segments very similar in structure to those of the viral oncogenes. At first this seemed unbelievable. Completely healthy people possess families of genes that cause cancer. This made no sense. It was then realised that the function of these genes was not to give us cancer, but to control all sorts of fundamental biological processes such as how cells become specialised in their functions, how an embryo grows, and how a wound repairs. Experiments showed that, when produced in excess, these genes can result in the cell stimulation that we see in cancer.

In fact, the whole oncogene system resembles a series of cog-wheels of growth control, transmitting information from outside the cell, through the cell membrane and down to the cell's 'brain' in the nucleus. Some are growth factors acting on receptors on other cells; others are the receptors themselves sitting in the cell membrane receiving signals from the outside world telling them how to behave. Still others are small cogs in the control pathways from membrane to nucleus. In the last twelve months, a whole new family of oncogenes responsible for deciding when a gene will make a protein have been discovered – the transcription factors.

The system is incredibly complex, but at least a complete understanding of cancer at a molecular level is now a realistic prospect. We can see how things can go wrong: a growth factor may be produced in excess quantities; a receptor may alter in such a way that it no longer needs a signal to stimulate growth. A myriad of changes can occur at the molecular level resulting in a tumour. This explains why cancer behaves so differently in different patients. An analysis of those changes could have profound significance for the way in which we treat cancer.

Oncogenes in diagnosis

Although this area of research is very young, there are already hints of considerable progress in relating tumour behaviour to its molecular make-up. A good example is the gene c-erbB2 in breast cancer. In around 40 per cent of women with breast cancer, the molecular make-up of the tumour shows subtle changes which can be measured at the time they have surgery. If the c-erbB2 gene is increased either within the DNA or in the amount of protein that it makes, then the overall outlook for that patient is much poorer. This type of information can be very useful in deciding which patients also need chemotherapy. Because many treatments have unpleasant side effects, they should preferably be given only to those patients who need them, and not to those who do not.

In the near future we may also be able to make very accurate predictions about who is likely to get cancer. We now know some of the molecular disturbances that cause cancer. It may be possible to predict whether people are likely to get the disease by examining their genetic material at a specific site. If you knew that your chances of dying with lung cancer were going to be 100 per cent if you smoked, but only 10 per cent if you did not, it could change your views on smoking. There may be other ways in which we can predict the likelihood of specific cancer types emerging and so take appropriate action, such as dietary and environmental control. Furthermore, it would allow us to target screening programmes specifically on people at greatest risk. One dilemma in screening is the sheer numbers involved. With breast cancer, for example, it is not just the time and effort required to pick up a single tumour, but also the risk of repeated mammography on the normal breast. If we could predict the likelihood of a woman developing breast cancer by examining her genetic make-up, the whole screening process could be streamlined.

Can oncogenes be tampered with to eradicate a tumour? The first hints that this may be possible are now emerging. There are several ways of inhibiting the function of an oncogene. For example, molecules can be constructed that block the proteins which stimulate cell growth. This type of strategy has been used in drug design in other areas of medicine and can be very effective. Of course these developments may have profound consequences for normal cells and we will have to learn how to use new drugs selectively. But here is a system which offers considerable hope for future developments.

CENTRES OF EXCELLENCE

One of the problems facing us in cancer treatment, is how best to use the resources we have. Ideally, all hospitals should have some form of cancer treatment service and this is true to some extent. But at a time when treatment is changing, it makes good sense to concentrate expensive resources in such a way that all can benefit from them. One way of doing this is to create cancer centres, usually in larger towns associated with a university medical school. This means the cancer centre benefits from the research and teaching atmosphere in which ideas can be questioned and discussed and research programmes instigated.

The problem then becomes how to get the patient to the centre. In Scotland an ideal situation has evolved with just four cancer centres in Edinburgh, Glasgow, Aberdeen and Dundee. Specialists from these centres go out to clinics in many general hospitals on a weekly basis to see new patients and follow-up those who have been treated. In England the position is rather different. There are over fifty centres involved in cancer treatment which have radiotherapy facilities. Expertise in some of the smaller centres is very limited, and yet patients are only infrequently referred to the larger centres. Few doctors like to admit that they are unable to cope with a specific cancer type. Of course, going to a larger centre for treatment means inconvenience and disturbance, especially for patients not used to travelling. We badly need better organisation in the provision of cancer services in England. There are many political problems in doing so. No politician wants to be seen standing idly by whilst a small cancer centre is closed. For this reason, attempts to rationalise cancer treatment in London, where there are over twenty units currently operating, have failed. It will be interesting to see whether the proposals in the Government's white paper 'Working for Patients' result in any change.

For the time being how can you make sure of getting the best? It is very difficult to put together a 'Good Cancer Centre Guide' because there are so many factors involved. For example, an elderly person with a small and easily curable skin cancer may be treated just as well in a small and relatively poorly equipped centre. But for more complex treatment the facilities and expertise available may be totally inadequate. We have put together some of the features of a good centre, so you at least have something to go by. But if you are worried about anything the most important thing is to ask to see the consultant and discuss things.

A GOOD CANCER CENTRE

- Is part of a major hospital with full backup facilities in many specialities.
- Is carrying out research to assess new cancer treatments.
- Is involved in the teaching of doctors, nurses, physicists, radiographers in cancer treatment.
- Has adequate facilities for radiotherapy including at least two linear accelerators, simulator and full planning computer facilities.
- Has specialists in medical oncology (chemotherapy) on its staff.
- Has councelling services to help with any problems you may have.

CANCER CHARITIES

In the appendix, the various cancer charities, together with their addresses and telephone numbers, are listed. What is the best way to choose which one to donate to? Although clearly they all aim to improve the treatment of cancer, they have different philosophies and different methods of organisation. As charities, they all face the same problems of collecting money, and have evolved similar strategies with a network of local appeal directors and voluntary helpers. Many operate shops which sell high quality goods and the profit, in turn, is ploughed into cancer research.

The largest is the Imperial Cancer Research Fund, which collects around £28 million annually. It has one main laboratory next to the Royal College of Surgeons in Lincoln's Inn Fields, London, and a smaller laboratory at Clare Hall in the suburbs of north London. It also has a variety of units and groups scattered around British hospitals and universities. It has a very cohesive scientific policy, firmly based in exploiting recent advances in our understanding of the molecules that make up a living cell and how they can go wrong. In addition, it funds a whole range of other cancer research activities, from evaluating complementary medicine through to studying the causes of cancer.

The second biggest charity is the Cancer Research Campaign. Rather than having its own laboratories, it identifies projects from proposals submitted from universities and hospitals throughout the country. Various committees select the best of these proposals and fund them according to their quality. Such committees, composed of senior cancer researchers and doctors, tend to be very conservative. Imaginative proposals from brilliant young investigators may not get the reception they deserve compared with more conventional projects which are less likely to produce major breakthroughs. Many of the projects are relatively small, with maybe just one staff member. This does allow the Cancer Research Campaign to fund projects throughout the UK.

One of the major problems for both charities is how to decide what to do next. The cynic's view of cancer research is that any research proposal either cannot be done or has been done before. Such nihilistic views are surprisingly common in many of the committees which control cancer research funding. Many research groups raise their own funds directly. Those associated with a hospital are often given money by grateful patients or their relatives and sometimes are left money in wills. This type of bequest is often useful to get new projects started and gives the investigator, rather than an anonymous committee, financial control. Like all spheres of human activity, there are political forces at work in determining who controls the flow of cash at any time.

Several factors may help you to decide how to go about giving money for cancer research. The first may be the presence of a particular organisation locally. If there is a charity shop or local organiser, they may well be able to advise you. If you want to know how the money will be spent, ask for the charity's annual report. All provide a detailed and informative report of their activities.

If you are scientifically inclined, then the scientific report will provide a short summary of each project being carried out. By using this book, you will get an overview of the cancer problem and you may be able to form your own opinion about the likelihood of success of a single charity's portfolio of research.

Dealing with local charities is much more difficult as, of course, they do not have the resources or expertise to be very professional about their fund-raising. Funding cancer research is like the stock exchange. The larger cancer charities are like the unit trusts having shares in a multitude of projects, some of which may well bite the dust while others may become major breakthroughs. Smaller, local charities stand or fall by the quality of their research and the ideas behind them. There may be less of a track record. These risky shares might produce high dividends; only those involved can tell you. If you are proposing to give money, do not hesitate to find out exactly what it is going on. If you are worried about the quality of the project, you may ask why the researchers have not asked for a grant from one of the major charities. There may be good reasons for this: it may be a pilot project, or one only appropriate to a particular area of the country. On the whole, however, good research groups tend to get funding from the major charities as well as local grants. Other sources of funding for cancer research come from the Government's Medical Research Council (MRC). However, because of the unique nature of funding from cancer charities, MRC support has dwindled at times of recession in the research world as a whole. The Department of Health also have various schemes to fund clinically oriented cancer research, especially concerning the logistics of cancer care.

Cancer research is surprisingly expensive. The equipment and staff for the laboratory of a single scientist entering the most productive period of his career at the age of about thirty, will cost a quarter of a million pounds. In addition, £100 000 per year running expenses will be needed. But it is only by doing this that the developments we have already seen have occurred.

Looking into the crystal ball to see how cancer treatment will change is difficult. It is unlikely that there will suddenly be a magic pill to correct the growth abnormality of cancer. Instead as we learn more about the molecules of life, the process of cancer will be more clearly understood. Then drugs will be developed to selectively control deviant cells as they grow. Research, first in the laboratory and then at the bedside, will produce the cancer treatments for the twenty-first century.

GETTING THE FACTS

FURTHER READING LIST

GENERAL

BRYAN, J. AND LYALL, J. *Living with cancer* Penguin, 1987. op.
Written by two journalists who have contributed to several health publications. Contributions from famous individuals who have had cancer. This, coupled with good practical advice, makes the book a supportive one, though medical facts are a little thin on the ground and the attention to specific types of cancer makes much of it irrelevant to most readers.

DOBREE, C. *Cancer* Ebury Press, 1988. op.
This book is one in a medical series written by a GP. It is laid out as a series of questions with long paragraphs as replies. These come under rather loosely defined chapters and looking for specific facts may be difficult.

SCOTT, R. B. *Cancer: the facts* Oxford University Press, 1980.
This is part of a series of books published by OUP, two of which are about cancer. The main drawback is that it is now a little out of date.

SMEDLEY, H., SIKORA, K. AND STEPNEY, R. *Cancer: what it is and how it's treated* B. Blackwell, 1985.
Written by two cancer specialists and a medical journalist. The book has a good scientific basis and there is an emphasis on treatment.

WILLIAMS, C. J. AND WILLIAMS, S. *Cancer: a guide to patients and their families* Wiley, 1986.
Written by a cancer specialist and his wife (a physiotherapist). A book with very many short chapters. Thirty-five out of fifty-four chapters are devoted to specific cancers and therefore much of the information in the book will be irrelevant to many people.

PREVENTION

DOLL, R. AND PETO, R. *Causes of cancer* Oxford University Press, 1982.

DOYAL, L. AND EPSTEIN, S. S. *Cancer in Britain: the politics of prevention* Pluto Press, 1983. op.

GOODWIN, P. *Can you avoid cancer?* BBC, 1984.

WHELAN, E. *Preventing cancer* Sphere, 1980. op.

SPECIFIC DISEASES

The British Association of Cancer United Patients (BACUP) provides excellent small booklets on specific diseases and types of cancer treatment which are very helpful and may be more up-to-date than some of the books listed below.

Breast cancer

BAUM, M. *Breast cancer: the facts* Oxford University Press, 1981; 1988.

FAULDER, C. *Breast cancer* Virago, 1982.

Colonic cancer

SCHINDLER, M. *Living with a colostomy: practical advice on overcoming the problems* Turnstone Press, 1985.

Childhood cancers

BAKER, L. S. *You and leukaemia: a day at a time* Saunders, 1978.

PARKER, M. AND MAUGER D. *Children with cancer: a handbook for families and helpers* Cassell, 1979. op.

Lung cancer

WILLIAMS, C. J. *Lung cancer: the facts* Oxford University Press, 1984.

COMPLEMENTARY THERAPY

Some of these books are a little extreme, advocating a strict diet which has no real basis. Some exaggerate the benefits of complementary therapies which should only be regarded as an adjunct to orthodox medicine.

BISHOP, B. *A time to heal* Severn House, 1985.

BROHN, P. *The Bristol Programme* Century, 1987.

BROHN, P. *Gentle giants: the powerful story of one woman's unconventional struggle against breast cancer* Century, 1986.

CAPRA, F. *The turning point* Fontana, 1983.

CHAITOW, L. *About laetrils: vitamin B17 and the fight against cancer* Thorsons, 1979. op.

CHAITOW, L. *An end to cancer? the nutritional approach to its prevention and control* Thorsons, 1983. op.

CONSUMERS' ASSOCIATION *Patient's guide to the National Health* Consumers' Association, 1983. op.

COUSINS, N. *Anatomy of an illness as perceived by the patient* Bantam, 1987. op.

GARDNER, M. J. *et al eds The atlas of cancer mortality in England and Wales, 1968–78* Wiley, 1983.

GURALNICK, E. AND LEVITT, P. M. *The cancer reference book* Harper & Row, 1984.

HARVEY, D. *The power to heal* Aquarian Press, 1983. op.

HOFFMAN, D. *The holistic herbal* Element, 1988. op.

HOLMES, D. *New hope and improved treatment for cancer patients* Wiley, 1982.

INGLIS, B. AND WEST R. *The alternative health guide* M. Joseph, 1984.

INGLIS, B. *The diseases of civilisation* Granada, 1983.

KOTHARI, M. L. AND METHA, L. A. *Cancer: myths and realities* M. Boyars, 1979.

LAWRENCE, F. ED *Additives: your complete survival guide* Century, 1986. op.

LESHAN, L. *How to meditate: a guide to self discovery* Turnstone Press, 1983.

LESHAN, L. *You can fight for your life* Thorsons, 1984. op.

MORRA, M. AND POTTS, E. *Choices* Avon, 1980. op.

NATIONAL CONSUMER COUNCIL *Patients' rights* National Consumer Council, 1983. op.

PEARCE, I. C. B. *The holistic approach to cancer* Findlay, 1983. op.

RICHARDS, D. *The topic of cancer: when the killing has to stop* Pergamon Press, 1982. op.

SARTON, M. *A reckoning* Women's Press, 1984.

SCALA, J. *Making the vitamin connection* Harper & Row, 1985. op.

SIMONTON, O. C. *Getting well again* Bantam, 1980. op.

WEATHERHEAD, L. *The Christian agnostic* Hodder & Stoughton, 1967. op.

AFTER TREATMENT

HINTON, J. *Dying* Penguin, 1971.

KUBLER-ROSS, E. *Living with death and dying* Souvenir Press, 1982.

LAMPEN, D. *Facing death* Quaker Home Service, 1979.

LAMERTON, R. *Care of the dying* Penguin, 1980.

PARKES, C. M. *Bereavement: studies of grief in adult life* Tavistock; Penguin, 1986.

SAUNDERS, C. M. *ed The management of terminal malignant disease* E. Arnold, 1984.

PERSONAL VIEW

ANDERSON, G. *It happened to me* Futura, 1986.

BURTON, L. *Care of the child facing death* Routledge, 1974. op.

CHAMPION, B. AND POWELL, J. *Champion's story* Fontana, 1982.

DE BEAUVOIR, S. *A very easy death* Penguin, 1969.

GIBRAN, K. *The prophet* Heinemann, 1926; 1972; Pan, 1980.

GRAHAM, J. *In the company of others: understanding the human needs of cancer patients* Gollancz, 1983. op.

GREEN, W. *The long road home* Lion, 1985; pbk, 1986.

HELMAN, E. *An autumn life: how a surgeon faces his fatal illness* Faber, 1986.

KUBLER-ROSS, E. *Death: the final stage of growth* Prentice Hall, 1975. op.

LAMERTON, R. *East End doc* Lutterworth, 1986.

LEWIS, C. S. *A grief observed* Faber, 1966.

PIFF, C. *Let's face it* Gollancz, 1985; Sphere, 1986. op.

SHAW, G. B. *The doctor's dilemma* Longman, Green, 1957. op.

USEFUL ADDRESSES

CANCER INFORMATION SERVICES

British Association of Cancer United
Patients (BACUP)
  121/123 Charterhouse Street
  London EC1M 6AA
  ☎ 01 608 1661
  Freephone outside London:
  0800 181199
CARE: Cancer and Aftercare
  21 Zetland Road
  Redland
  Bristol BS6 7AH
  ☎ 0272 427419
CancerLink
  17 Britannia Street
  London WC1X 9JN
  ☎ 01 833 2451
New Approaches to Cancer
  c/o Park Attwood Clinic
  Trimpley
  Bewdley
  Worcs. DY12 1RE
  ☎ 0299 7375

COMPLEMENTARY MEDICINE CONTACTS

Anthroposophical Society in Great
Britain
  Rudolf Steiner House
  35 Park Road
  London NW1 6XT
  ☎ 01 723 4400
    01 723 8219

Association of Humanistic Psychology
in Britain
  5 Leyton Road
  London N1
  ☎ 01 226 4240
Association of Hypnotists and
Psychotherapists
  12 Cross Street
  Nelson, Lancs. BB9 7EN
  ☎ 0282 699378
Dr Edward Bach Centre
  Mount Vernon
  Sotwell, Wallingford
  Oxon. OX10 0PZ
  ☎ 0491 39489
British Association of Art Therapists
  13c Northwood Road
  London N6 5TL
British Homeopathic Association
  27a Devonshire Street
  London W1N 1RJ
  ☎ 01 935 2163
British Medical Acupuncture Society
  67/69 Chancery Lane
  London WC2A 1AF
British Wheel of Yoga
  1 Hamilton Place
  Boston Road
  Sleaford
  Lincs. NG34 7ES
  ☎ 0529 306851
Council for Acupuncture
  Panther House
  38 Mount Pleasant
  London WC1X 0AP
  ☎ 01 837 8026

Friends of Shanti Nilaya
  PO Box 212
  London NW8 7NW
  (based on Elizabeth Kubler-Ross)
Institute for Complementary Medicine
  21 Portland Place
  London WIN 3AF
  (Send SAE: can supply names and
  addresses of local individuals in
  various branches of complementary
  medicine.)
  ☎ 01 636 9543
Matthew Manning Centre
  39 Abbeygate Street
  Bury St Edmunds
  Suffolk IP33 1LW
  ☎ 0284 769502
National Federation of Spiritual
Healers
  Old Manor Farm Studio
  Church Street
  Sunbury-on-Thames
  Middx. TW16 6RG
  ☎ 09327 83164/5
National Institute of Medical
Herbalists
  Secretary: PO Box 3
  41 Hatherley Road
  Winchester
  Hants. SO22 6RR
  ☎ 0962 68776
The Royal London Homeopathic
Hospital
  Great Ormond Street
  London WC1 3HR
  ☎ 01 837 3091
    01 837 8833

Society of Homeopaths
  2 Artizan Road
  Northampton NN1 4HU
  ☎ 0604 21400
Society of Teachers of the Alexander
Technique
  10 London House
  266 Fulham Road
  London SW10 9EL
  ☎ 01 351 0828

COMPLEMENTARY CANCER CENTRES

Auchenkyle Health Clinic
  Southwoods Road
  Troon
  Ayrshire KA10 7EL
  ☎ 0292 311414
Bournemouth Centre of
Complementary Medicine
  26 Sea Road
  Boscombe, Bournemouth
  Dorset BH5 1DF
  ☎ 0202 36354
Bristol Cancer Help Centre
  Grove House
  Cornwallis Grove
  Bristol BS8 4PG
  ☎ 0272 743216
The Health Education Authority
  Hamilton House
  Mabledon Place
  London WC1H 9TX
  ☎ 01 631 0930
Morecambe Bay Cancer Help Centre
  Secretary: Mrs Janet Stewart
  11 College Road
  Windermere
  Cumbria LA23 1BU
  ☎ 09662 2548

Wessex Cancer Help Centre
8 South Street
Chichester
West Sussex PO19 1EH
☎ 0243 778516

SELF-HELP AND SUPPORT GROUPS

Action on Smoking and Health
5–11 Mortimer Street
London W1N 7RH
☎ 01 637 9843
Breast Care and Mastectomy
Association
26a Harrison Street
London WC1H 8JG
☎ 01 837 0908
Colostomy Welfare Group
38–39 Eccleston Square
London SW1V 1PB
☎ 01 828 5175
Compassionate Friends
6 Denmark Street
Bristol BS1 5DQ
☎ 0272 292778
CRUSE: Bereavement Care
CRUSE House
126 Sheen Road
Richmond
Surrey TW9 1UR
☎ 01 940 4818
Ileostomy Association of Great Britain
and Ireland
Central Office
Amblehurst House
Black Scotch Lane
Notts. NG18 PF
☎ 0623 28099

Impaired Lives Insurance Bureau
Trevone House
Pannells Court
Guildford
Surrey GU1 4EY
☎ 0483 575282
The Leukaemia Care Society
PO Box 82
Exeter
Devon EX2 5DP
☎ 0392 218514
Leukaemia Research Fund
43 Great Ormond Street
London WC1N 3JJ
☎ 01 405 0101
MacMillan Nurses
Anchor House
15–19 Britten Street
London SW3 3TZ
☎ 01 351 7811
National Association of Laryngectomee
Clubs
39 Eccleston Square
London SW1V 1PB
☎ 01 834 2857
National Carers Association
29 Chilworth Mews
London W2 3RG
☎ 01 724 7776
Neuroblastoma Society
Mrs J. Oldridge
Woodlands
Ordsall Park Road
Retford
Notts. DN22 7PJ
☎ 0777 709238

Society for the Prevention of
Asbestosis and Industrial Diseases
  38 Drapers Road, Enfield
  Middx. EN2 8LU
  ☎ 01 366 1640
Stoma Advisory Service
  Abbot Laboratories
  Queenborough, Kent
  ☎ 0795 580099
Tenovus Breast Cancer Information
Centre
  College Building
  University Place, Splott
  Cardiff CF1 1SA
  ☎ 0222 483500
Urostomy Association
  Mrs Angela Cook
  Buckland, Beaumont Park
  Danbury, Essex CM3 4DE
  ☎ 024 541 4294
Women's National Cancer Control
Campaign
  1 South Audley Street
  London W1Y 5DQ
  ☎ 01 499 7532

CANCER CHARITIES

Cancer Research Campaign
  2 Carlton House Terrace
  London SW1Y 5AR
  ☎ 01 930 8972
Imperial Cancer Research Fund
  44 Lincoln's Inn Fields
  London WC2A 3PX
  ☎ 01 242 0200

International School for Cancer Care
  Royal Marsden Hospital
  Fulham Road
  London SW3 6JJ
  ☎ 01 352 8171, ext. 2305
  Oxford (0865) 67123
Malcolm Sargent Cancer Fund for
Children
  14 Abingdon Road
  London W8 6AF
  ☎ 01 937 4548
Marie Curie Memorial Foundation
  28 Belgrave Square
  London SW1X 8QG
  ☎ 01 235 3325
Sue Ryder Foundation
  Sue Ryder Home
  Cavendish, nr Sudbury
  Suffolk CO10 8AY
  ☎ 0787 280252
Tenovus Institute
  111 Cathedral Road
  Cardiff CF1 9PF
  ☎ 0222 342851
Wallace Kingston Trust for Abdominal
Diseases
  The Drove
  Fuzzy Drove
  Basingstoke
  Hants. RG22 3LU
  ☎ 0256 52320

GLOSSARY

ANALGESIC a drug that relieves pain

BENIGN abnormal growth in a tissue that does not spread or invade surrounding organs

BIOPSY removal of a small piece of tissue to make a diagnosis by examining it under the microscope

CARCINOGEN a chemical that causes cancer

CARCINOMA a cancer that arises from cells in one of the lining tissues inside the breast, lung, skin or many other sites

CHEMOTHERAPY the use of drugs to treat disease including cancer

COLOSTOMY an opening in the front of the abdomen to divert the contents of the bowel after removal of the rectum

CT SCAN computerised tomography scan – a series of X-rays which, when analysed by a powerful computer, provide very clear images of internal organs

DNA deoxyribonucleic acid – the thread of life which contains genes and is found in the nucleus of the cell

ENDOSCOPY looking inside the body with a fine tube to see if all is well

GENE one of a series of units of information in DNA

GRADING determining how a tumour is likely to behave by looking at it down the microscope

HEPATOMA a tumour arising in the liver

HEMIBODY radiotherapy given to half the body – a useful way of relieving pain in patients who have widespread cancer

HIV human immunodeficiency virus – the cause of AIDS

HORMONE THERAPY treatment of cancer by hormones – naturally produced chemicals involved in controlling various organs

INTRACAVITARY a type of radiotherapy in which a radioactive material is placed into a body cavity – most commonly the uterus

INTERSTITIAL a type of radiotherapy which involves placing of radioactive wires directly into a tumour whilst the patient is anaesthetised

INVASIVE a cancer that is penetrating surrounding normal tissues and is in the process of spreading

LEUKAEMIA a cancer arising from the blood-forming cells of the bone marrow or lymph nodes

MALIGNANT abnormal growths that spread by invasion and by the blood and lymphatic system

MAMMOGRAM examination of the breast by X-ray

MASS a swelling or lump

MASTECTOMY removal of the breast

MELANOMA a type of skin cancer which contains pigment cells

METASTASIS the spreading of a malignant tumour from the site in which it started to other parts of the body

NUCLEUS the 'brains' of the cell – where all its activity is coordinated

ONCOLOGY the branch of medicine involving the study of tumours

PALLIATION the relief of symptoms without necessarily curing the illness

PRIMARY TUMOUR the original tumour before any spread has occurred

RADIOTHERAPY treatment with X-rays or radioactive materials

RADICAL treatment aimed to cure

SARCOMA a cancer arising from the body's connective tissue – e.g. muscle and bone

SCREENING examining people to pick up a disease early

SECONDARY TUMOUR a tumour which has spread or metastasised from the primary (original) site

STAGING the classification of a tumour depending on how far it has spread

TUMOUR an abnormal swelling or enlargement that is no use to the body

SYSTEMIC THERAPY treatment (usually drugs) that goes right round the body through the bloodstream

INDEX

THE HAMMERSMITH
CANCER CENTRE APPEAL

We urgently need to build a new Cancer Centre at Hammersmith Hospital. Our laboratories, generously funded by the Imperial Cancer Research Fund, are excellent, but our treatment facilities are lagging behind. Treatments that belong to the twenty-first century are carried out in conditions firmly rooted in the nineteenth. A former Victorian workhouse is home to the wards, the Radiotherapy Department is a long walk from the outpatients clinic and we lack a treatment centre that caters for the unique needs of cancer patients.

So what is planned is an exciting new development. The building will cost £13 million. It will help us to help over 5000 patients a year. The Appeal's contribution is £5 million and has to be raised with your help and the remainder will come from government and commercial sources.

But we are asking you to contribute to more than bricks and mortar. This is a radical project with a revolutionary approach. For the first time, holistic therapies will be available alongside conventional treatment.

If you would like further details of the appeal, please contact the Appeal Director at the address below or telephone (01) 743 9655.

With your support, we can 'Help Hammer Cancer'. Please give generously – we need your help!

To: The Hammersmith Cancer Centre Appeal
        Du Cane Road, London W12 0NN

I/WE WISH TO MAKE A DONATION TO THE HAMMERSMITH CANCER CENTRE APPEAL. PLEASE FIND ENCLOSED A CHEQUE FOR £....... MADE PAYABLE TO 'RPMS CANCER TRUST'.

NAME_____

ADDRESS_____

REGISTERED CHARITY NO. 299907
£8 million will come from government and commercial sources